Homoeopathy for the Primary Health Care Team

A Guide for GPs, Midwives, District Nurses and Other Health Professionals

Paul Downey
MBChB MRCGP MFHom HMD DCH DRCOG

BUTTERWORTH
HEINEMANN

[redacted]

To
Mum and Dad
Kelly
Hannah, Harriet and Patrick

Butterworth-Heinemann
Linacre House, Jordan Hill, Oxford OX2 8DP
A division of Reed Educational and Professional Publishing Ltd

A member of the Reed Elsevier plc group

OXFORD BOSTON JOHANNESBURG
MELBOURNE NEW DELHI SINGAPORE

First published 1997

British Library Cataloguing in Publication Data
A catalogue record for this book is available from the British Library

Library of Congress Cataloguing in Publication Data
A catalogue record for this book is available from the Library of Congress

ISBN 0 7506 2999 1

Typeset by E & M Graphics, Midsomer Norton, Bath
Printed and bound in Great Britain by Biddles Ltd, Guildford and King's Lynn

Contents

Section 4 Homoeopathy and the Community Health Care Team

Section 5 Materia Medica

Introduction

There is a growing interest in complementary medicine amongst both the public and the medical and nursing professions. I believe that general practice is the ideal setting where many of these therapies can be utilized and where we can try and evaluate and integrate the most useful treatments into daily care.

Each year 280 million people are seen in the primary care setting: for 90% of people, this is their only contact with the health service.[1]

Homoeopathy is essentially a therapy for the individual and that will always remain the basic philosophy. This does not mean that it cannot be tried and tested in the primary care setting, and used to complement other therapeutic approaches.

This book has been written for those working in primary care. I have tried to provide a logical introduction to homoeopathic medicine. I have written from the perspective of someone who has read many texts on the subject over the years, but never found one that covered all the concepts a beginner needs to understand. I hope it achieves that aim. I do not pretend to be an expert. As in other disciplines of health care, one is continually learning.

The study of homoeopathy is potentially very rewarding. Whether one is reading about the subject from curiosity or beginning more detailed research, there is plenty to learn.

The growth in public interest in complementary medicine requires those working in primary care to have a least a working knowledge of the systems so that they can give an informed opinion to patients.

My own interest in homoeopathy began whilst I was an undergraduate. Fortunately, in Liverpool where I trained there has been a strong tradition of homoeopathy for over a century, complemented by an active homoeopathic hospital. Thus I took my first tentative steps down this particular road.

The study of homoeopathy blends other disciplines such as botany, medical history, herbal medicine, medical philosophy and toxicology. Such a vast array of topics can only be integrated by years of study. However, this does not preclude the interested beginner from grasping the fundamentals of the subject, and beginning to use this knowledge in the primary care setting at a basic level.

Primary care has seen major changes in its workload in the last 10 years. The modern GP has proved adaptable in learning new skills and offering new treatments to patients. The other members of the team, including practice nurses, district nurses and health visitors, are all extending their roles as health care delivery evolves.

I believe it would be relatively easy for interested practitioners, be they doctors or nurses, to integrate homoeopathy into everyday practice with a basic understanding of homoeopathic philosophy and the medicines used. Homoeopathic medicines are considerably cheaper than other medicines and their use has the potential to provide a means of reducing overall drug costs,[2] as well as avoiding the side-effects of some of today's more powerful drugs.

When asked to prepare a text I had to consider what I would achieve by writing another textbook on the subject. After consideration, it occurred to me that, despite the huge range of works available, there is not one that addresses the issue from the primary health care viewpoint.

Is this important? I believe so. There is in my experience as a GP tutor and GP course organizer a growing interest in the subject amongst younger doctors and health professionals prepared to open their minds to ideas that differ from the traditional models of medical therapy. At the same time there is a growing demand from doctors, nurses, midwives and health visitors for more information and courses about homoeopathy.

When I began to think about the format of this book I felt it would be useful to provide in one volume an outline of the development of homoeopathy to the present day, with particular reference to its rise in the UK. Whilst studying for the MFHom examination, I was aware of some of the gaps in current texts and that no one text covered all aspects of the topic. Whilst this book is designed to give the complete newcomer an easy-to-read introduction, I hope it will also be a useful reference for those contemplating more advanced study.

The book is designed to tackle conditions commonly seen in general practice, and for that I make no apologies. The conditions mentioned are not exhaustive, and I believe only time, experience and discussion with other homoeopaths can expand a practitioner's expertise.

Currently in the UK homoeopathy is enjoying a resurgence of popularity. Due to insufficient numbers of medical practitioners, many practitioners are non-medically qualified (NMQP) and, with some exceptions, namely those registered with the RSHom, the practice of homoeopathy is still unregulated in many cases.

It is estimated that homoeopathy is the third most popular form of complementary medicine after manipulative therapies and acupuncture.

However, accurate figures for the true number of consultations taking place are not available.

A study in Oxford in 1986 (Anderson and Anderson, 1993) estimated that, of 200 GPs, 38% had some training in a form of complementary medicine. Homoeopathy was found to be an acceptable form of therapy by 47% of respondents, and 70% thought it should be available on the National Health Service.[3]

However, a General Medical Services Committee survey in 1992 found that only 19% of respondents thought homoeopathy should be available in surgery – a massive 50% thought it should not.

A survey of GPs in the magazine *Doctor* in 1992 found that 80% of GPs replying thought that homoeopathy was effective.[4]

A recent survey of nurses showed that 58% of respondents had used or recommended a form of complementary therapy. Of those practising, the majority used some form of therapy involving touch, massage or aromatherapy, which seems logical in view of the close physical contact nurses have with patients on a daily basis. Some 25% of those using therapies identified homoeopathy as a subject they would like to learn more about, and 12% were looking at further training in the subject.[5]

Homoeopathy, like other therapies, has seen a resurgence in the last two decades. The reasons for this are many and include the growing discontent amongst the public about the use of powerful medicines and their side-effects, the increasing beliefs that 'natural is better', and a shift in patient attitudes – greater patient interest in health issues and personal well-being. It seems appropriate that its resurgence should coincide with the two-hundreth anniversary of the first description of homoeopathy in 1796 and with the height of its popularity at the end of the last century.

References

1. *Royal College of General Practitioners Information Fact Sheet* no 3 July 1995.
2. Swayne J. The cost and effectiveness of homoeopathy. *Br Hom J* 1992; **81**: 148–150.
3. Anderson E, Anderson P. General practitioners and alternative medicine. *Br J Gen Pract* 1993; **43**: 232–235.
4. *Doctor* 16th July 1992.
5. Alternative update. A true complement? *Nursing Times* Jan–Feb 1996; **92**: no. 5 (survey).

Section 1

An Introduction to the History and Philosophy of Homoeopathy

1

Definitions of homoeopathic terms

I once read that the word 'jargon' could be defined as 'the technical language of another discipline'.

Certainly for those first encountering homoeopathy there is much in the terminology that needs to be defined. The following list should help.

Homoeopathy	from the Greek *homoios*, meaning like, and *pathos*, meaning suffering
Constitution	the sum of the totality of the patient's symptoms, temperament and appearance, which are important in choosing a remedy in the classical way
Repertory	a book which contains a list of symptoms or *rubrics*, which are cross-referenced with all the remedies which may correspond with those symptoms
Materia medica	a listing of remedies and their corresponding symptom pictures
Vital force	the energy of a living system responsible for the state of health
Potency	the homoeopathic strength of a remedy, denoted by symbols X, C or M. Potency is paradoxically more effective in higher dilution as the preparation of the remedy has energized the medicine to a greater degree
Polychrest	about 30–40 remedies are used very frequently. They not only fit constitutional types but also have a wide range of specific applications
Modality	this refers to factors which influence a symptom, i.e. make it worse or better, such as the effect of heat on certain patient symptoms. The symbols < and > denote when a modality improves (>) or worsens a symptom (<)
Nosodes	remedies derived from diseased tissue, or organisms. Isodes are remedies derived from the patient, and sarcodes are derived from animal organs

Proving	from the German *prufen*; this originates from the experiments originally carried out on healthy volunteers to record the symptoms induced by particular remedies
Aggravation	there are two types of aggravation: • *homoeopathic aggravation*, where the symptoms may temporarily worsen when taking a remedy, but then the patient improves • *disease aggravation*, where the patient's condition deteriorates because of the illness and an incorrect choice of remedy

2

A brief history of homoeopathy

Homoeopathy is a therapeutic method that involves the use of specially prepared and diluted medicinal substances. The medicines are chosen according to the patient's individual needs. Determining the exact match of remedy and patient can be difficult, but can be learnt with patience and study.

The word homoeopathy derives from the Greek words *homoios*, meaning like, and *pathos*, meaning suffering. The fundamental principle – like cures like – is that a substance that causes symptoms in a healthy person can, when those same symptoms occur in a sick person, help cure that patient by eliminating the disease.

No text on the subject of homoeopathy can be considered complete without an appreciation of Samuel Hahnemann, the founder of homoeopathy.

Born in 1755 in Meissen, Germany, Hahnemann was the son of a ceramics worker. Encouraged by his father, the young Hahnemann was a prodigious reader and by the age of 12 was able to speak Greek so well that he was teaching the language to classmates. His gift for languages was to be an important factor in his later discovery of homoeopathy. His academic talents did not go unnoticed, and with support from a master called Müller he was permitted to enter higher school to complete his education.

Eventually, at the age of 20 he was admitted to the University of Leipzig to study medicine. His language skills enabled him to supplement his meagre funds to continue his education by translating major scientific works into German. In this way he became interested in many disciplines.

Dissatisfied with the medical teaching at Leipzig he transferred to Vienna. Poverty prevented him from completing his studies, but he was offered a post as medical adviser at Hermannstadt and during that time catalogued the library of Herr Brukenthal, the governor of Transylvania. During these 20 months he continued his medical studies. Eventually he presented his thesis and in 1779 he was awarded the title of Doctor of Medicine.

This was the beginning of a career that was to be characterized by frequent confrontations with his fellow professionals, several moves to other towns in search of work, raising a family and at the same time continuing his research and writing.

Hahnemann's first practice was in the mining town of Hettstedt where conditions were squalid. His criticism of the conditions tolerated by the occupants reveals a man who was already formulating ideas that today would be considered basic tenets of public health and disease transmission.

> I maintain that epidemics, in the beginning are largely illnesses of isolated individuals, which could easily be subjugated...if I omit unhealthy weather conditions, penury and poverty.

Thus, early on Hahnemann seems to be postulating the communicable nature of disease years ahead of the discoveries of Koch and Pasteur.

After 9 months he left for Dessau where he supplemented his income translating books. During this time he met and married his wife, Henriette.

Hahnemann moved on to the town of Gommern. Here he continued his translations of scientific texts, frequently adding comments of his own. His reputation in this field began to grow. He wrote an essay, 'Directions for curing old sores and indolent ulcers', in which he began his scathing attacks on the medical profession for their old-fashioned practices. Once more he elaborated his ideas on public health measures,such as public hygiene, fresh air and sensible diet.

The family's next move was to Dresden where Hahnemann met and worked with the chemist Antoine Lavoisier. It was at this time that Hahnemann discovered the first test for detecting arsenic poisoning. At this point in his career he abandoned medical practice because of his increasing disenchantment with the state of the medical treatments available.

Hahnemann was a locum medical officer of health in Dresden, and during this time his work included the supervision of prisons, as a result of which he became an advocate of prison reform.

Hahnemann next moved to Leipzig where his opposition to the accepted medical practices of bleeding and purging became so extreme that he published articles in newspapers decrying the treatments and those who practised them. He left Leipzig because of the 'unhealthy air' 7 years later.

During this period he began translating other scientific works, including in 1790 *Materia Medica* by William Cullen, professor of chemistry at Edinburgh University. In this treatise Cullen described the role played by cinchona and its effect in malaria (ague). Cullen argued that it achieved its therapeutic effect by acting as a tonic on the stomach.

Hahnemann, as was his practice when translating, annotated the book with his own thoughts, arguing that Cullen's logic was wrong.

Hahnemann then went on to describe the effect cinchona (china) had when he deliberately took doses of it himself: 'all those symptoms which to me are typical of intermittent fever...all made their appearance'.

It can be deduced that Hahnemann ascertained that symptoms produced by a medicine in healthy people could be used to antagonize the symptoms of people with a disease causing a similar symptom picture. Thus was born the concept elaborated on in later years, and this was the first proving of a medicine.

The concept of like treating like was not new: Hippocrates (460–350 BC) had advocated such a theory as 'By similar things a disease is produced and through the application of like it is cured'. Paracelsus (1493–1541) had also postulated such a theory: 'sames must be cured by sames'. The Danish physician Georg Stahl also stated: 'I am convinced that disease will yield to and be cured by remedies that produce similar affections'. However it was Hahnemann who was to be the first to develop a therapeutic system based on this philosophy.

It was to be 6 years before Hahnemann published his beliefs on the therapeutic system he was to call homoeopathy. During those years Hahenmann was to experiment on himself and friends and family, observing the effects of a number of possibly therapeutic substances.

Hahnemann certainly had time for these experiments. In 1792 he obtained the post of medical officer in a private nursing home in the castle at Georgenthal under the patronage of Duke Ernst von Sachsen-Gotha. The Duke had heard of Hahnemann's ideas and invited him to work at Georgenthal. However, his only patient was to be an author named Klockenbring whom Hahnemann rescued from the asylum and cured within 7 months. During the next 3 years he continued his wanderings, presumably persevering with his experiments, and in a 13-year timespan Hahnemann and his family moved 20 times. In 1796, whilst at Königslutter, Hahnemann published a paper describing his ideas on homoeopathy for the first time. The paper appeared in Hufeland's journal and was entitled 'Essay on a new principle for ascertaining the curative properties of drugs, and some examination of previous principles'. In this paper Hahnemann systematically reviewed the old medical methods. He also refuted the idea of treating opposites with opposites: *contraria contrariis*.

He finally introduced his new ideas: 'apply to the disease to be healed...that remedy which is able to stimulate another artificially produced disease as similar as possible, and the former will be healed. *Simila similibus*, likes with likes'.

Hahnemann began to look at the question of dosage and strength. He noted that higher material doses of substances could aggravate symptoms, but lower, more dilute doses were equally, if not more, effective. Reducing the dose by serial dilution was carried out to precise methods, to be discussed later.

Hahnemann developed a more comprehensive list of medicines, carrying out experiments known as provings, from the German *prufen*, to test.

Hahnemann's nomadic life continued throughout the early 1800s. In 1805 he produced a work describing the properties of 27 remedies, all tested on himself and volunteers.

It was in 1810 that his seminal work, the *Organon of Rational Healing*, better known as the *Organon*, was first published. This was the culmination of 20 years of experimentation and became the standard reference work for generations of homoeopaths. Between 1810 and 1843 there were to be six editions of the *Organon*, each elaborating on Hahnemann's earlier ideas. The fundamental principle was *simila similibus curentur* – let like be treated with like.

It is an interesting quirk of history that the final volume, the sixth (in which the most important changes were made), was not published until 1921. The impact this was to have was enormous, and if it had been produced earlier it may have influenced the thinking of other later great homoeopaths, such as Kent, who did not live to see the sixth volume.

Hahnemann settled in relative calm in Leipzig between 1811 and 1820. He failed in his attempts to set up a homoeopathic institute and so decided to obtain a teaching post at the university. In 1812 he delivered a dissertation on white hellebore. This was not a lecture on homoeopathy, as many had expected. His oratorial skills were undeniably successful. He obtained his professorship and began lecturing at the university.

Hahnemann's arrogant teaching style was considered unrestrained and insulting, as he attacked the deficiencies of conventional medicine. His classes became unpopular. His following numbered a mere handful and they became the nucleus of his provers, who volunteered to test the medicines.

His time at Leipzig saw the publication of six volumes of *Materia Medica Pura* between 1811 and 1821.

In 1812 homoeopathy was used effectively in the treatment of typhus. Napoleon's retreating army had been struck down with the disease, and spread the infection throughout Europe. Homoeopathy proved more effective than conventional remedies of the time, and its popularity and use spread.

By 1821 Hahnemann was on the move again. Local, probably jealous physicians had conspired against him to prevent him preparing his remedies. A patient of his, Prince Schwarzenberg of Austria, had died as a result of intemperate living; Hahnemann's opponents had taken the opportunity to seize on the prince's death as evidence of the failure of homoeopathy.

Hahnemann retreated to Coethen where, under the patronage of a patient of his, the Duke of Anhalt Coethen, he was allowed to prepare and dispense remedies without opposition. He remained there for 11 years, which were apparently amongst the most contented of his troubled life. During this time he published his work *Chronic Diseases*, which was to arouse much debate. This book, written during the latter years of his life, expounded the theory that many illnesses are the result of a taint, be it acquired or inherited. These miasmatic diseases – psora, sycosis and syphilis – were the basis for all human ills.

In 1831 a cholera epidemic swept across Europe. In many centres homoeopathy was used and the death rates were significantly less than those of the allopaths, although cynics may say this was the result of the common-sense measures of rehydration and rest that Hahnemann employed.

Whatever the previous success of homoeopathy, the epidemic ensured that its reputation spread further afield. It was during this epidemic and Hahnemann's subsequent writings that he postulated the existence of 'infinitely small living organisms...which most probably form the matter of cholera'.

In 1830 Hahnemann's wife Henriette died and in the next few years Hahnemann was less active in his work. However, that changed in 1834 when Hahnemann, now aged 79, met a young patient who was subsequently to sweep him off his feet. The woman, Marie Melanie d'Hervilly, was about 30. It is believed that she had arranged to see Hahnemann with the sole intention of eventually marrying him. This she did – within 3 months of their first encounter!

Melanie had great ambitions for her husband, despite his age. She persuaded him to give up his work in Coethen and move to Paris to set up a practice. This he eventually did. His international fame ensured a prosperous practice, with the more than willing support of Melanie, who it is believed was involved in the treatment of patients, although not medically qualified herself. There has been much criticism of Melanie's influence on the ageing Hahnemann, but it appears that he was devoted to her.

In 1843, after several respiratory infections, Hahnemann died. He was buried in an umarked and unattended grave. It was not until 1898 that he was buried at the expense of the American homoeopathic doctors in Père Lachaise cemetery with a fitting memorial.

Summary

1755	Samuel Hahnemann born Meissen, Germany
1779	Doctorate, University of Erlangen, Germany
1790	Translation of Cullen's *Materia Medica*. First thoughts on homoeopathic principle
1796	Essay outlining homoeopathic principles, Hufeland's journal
1810–1843	*Organon*, six editions
1811–1821	*Materia Medica Pura*, six volumes.
1828	Chronic diseases. Miasmatic theory
1834	Married Melanie d'Hervilly
1843	Died in Paris
1921	Sixth edition of *Organon* eventually published

References

1. Ruthven Mitchell G. *Homoeopathy*. London: WH Allen, 1975.
2. Cook T. *Samuel Hahnemann – His Life and Times*. Wellingborough: Thorsons, 1971.

3

Homoeopathic remedies: source and preparation

When considering using a homoeopathic remedy, one must first understand where the remedy originated, and how it was produced. This chapter briefly explains both the preparation and manufacture of homoeopathic medicines.

It is thought that there are about 3000 substances available to the homoeopath, compared with about 200 at the time of Hahnemann's death. They are virtually all derived from natural sources, including plants, animal materials and minerals. Biological sources are used for special medicines called nosodes.

Sources

The plant kingdom accounts for approximately 60% of all homoeopathic medicines. The medicine may be derived from the whole plant, but it is more usual for a particular part of the plant to be used.

Certain remedies, such as Pulsatilla, Aconite and Chamomilla are derived from the whole plant. Others, such as Rhus Tox, are derived from the leaves.

Ipecac and Bryonia are derived from the roots, whereas Nux Vomica and Ignatia are derived from the seeds of their respective plants. Allium Cepa and Colchicum are taken from the bulbs of the plant. More detailed information on the source of the medicine can be obtained from a good materia medica.

The animal kingdom is used to produce many well-known and widely used medicines. Apis Mel and Cantharis are derived from the whole of the honey bee and Spanish fly respectively. Sepia is the ink of the cuttlefish, and therapies such as Tarentula and Lachesis are derived from the venom of the animal.

The third main group of sources of remedies are the chemical elements and minerals. It is sometimes easier to consider these in subgroups of those remedies which are soluble in an alcohol/water mixture, and those which are insoluble.

Amongst the minerals there are many well-known substances, including silica, calc carb, Arsenicum Album and Natrum Mur.

The metal elements which are insoluble include remedies such as plumbum, aurum and stannum. Non-metal elements include sulphur and graphites.

The biological sources mentioned above are used mainly for the production of special remedies called *nosodes*. These may be derived from fresh healthy organs of animals, called *sarcodes*, extracts of diseased tissue, called nosodes, or extracts from the patient, called *isodes*. A special type of nosode, called the *bowel nosode*, contains extract of cultures of stool containing intestinal bacteria.

How is a homoeopathic remedy prepared?

The mother tincture is the homoeopathic remedy in its most concentrated form, sometimes denoted by the symbol φ (phi). From the mother tincture the remedy is prepared.

To prepare a mother tincture the substance has to be treated in a specific way to retain the therapeutic properties of the remedy. Guidelines were laid down by Hahnemann and are still adhered to today. Specific pharmacopoeias give instructions on good manufacturing practice.

To prepare the mother tincture the substance undergoes four processes:

1. Maceration.
2. Extraction.
3. Ageing.
4. Filtration.

Maceration

Maceration is self-explanatory. The substance is ground in varying alcohol strengths and filtered.

Extraction

Extraction involves treating the macerated material with ethanol and distilled water. This helps dissolve the therapeutic substances in the starting material.

Ageing

The suspension is then stored for a predetermined time, for it to age.

Filtration

The suspension is filtered once more to provide the final mother tincture.

Potentization

The process by which Hahnemann believed that a medicine acquired its therapeutic action is called potentization. Diluting the substance alone may have altered the therapeutic efficacy of a substance, but Hahnemann noted that when the mixture was *succussed* (shaken with impact), the therapeutic effect appeared to be enhanced.

I will describe the preparation of a potency series as an example. The *decimal* potencies are based on a dilution of 1 : 10. The *centisimal* potencies are based on a dilution of 1 : 100. The decimal series is denoted by Roman X – 1X, 2X, 3X, etc. The centisimal series is denoted by Roman C – 1C, 2C, 3C, etc.

Decimal series

To prepare a decimal potency, one part of mother tincture is mixed with nine parts of 20–30% mixture of alcohol and pure water, and succussed. This is the first decimal potency – 1X. One part of the 1X solution is taken and mixed with a further nine parts of the alcohol/water solution and succussed. This is the second decimal potency – 2X. The serial dilution is repeated to produce other potencies – 6X, 24X, etc.

Centisimal series

To prepare a centisimal series the above procedure is used; however, the mother tincture is mixed one part to 99 parts of the alcohol/water mixture, in a 1 : 100 ratio. This is the 1C potency. The process is repeated, with one part of the 1C potency further diluted in 99 ml of the alcohol/water mixture; each stage is accompanied by succussion.

The dilutions can be represented as follows:

Decimal	Centisimal
1X 1 : 10	1C 1 : 100
2X 1 : 100	2C 1 : 10 000
3X 1 : 1000	3C 1 : 1 000 000
4X 1 : 10 000	
6X 1 : 1 000 000	

It can be seen that 2C and 4X are the same dilution, but the number of succussions, which influences the potency, is different.

Millemisimal series

A further series of potencies, the *millemisimal series*, is based on a 1 : 1000 dilution ratio. In the Hahnemann method of preparing potencies each step required a new test tube and the process was time-consuming.

In 1832 a Russian, Korsakov, described a method in which the same container was used to prepare all potencies. He argued that, on emptying the container, sufficient liquid remained on the walls to be used for the next dilution. This method became adopted for potency preparations above 200C.

Trituration

This is the process by which potencies are produced in solid form from insoluble substances. First the material is mixed and ground with powdered lactose. One part of the active substance is ground with 99 parts of pure lactose. The grinding process lasts about 1 hour and this is the potentizing process. This can be repeated by taking one part of the ground substance and mixing it with a further 99 parts of lactose to produce the second potency. Sufficient grinding and dilution usually render the material soluble, with an alcohol/water mixture at about the 8X potency.

Manufacture

The manufacture of homoeopathic medicines is carried out according to strict principles laid down by Hahnemann.

The larger companies, such as Weleda, are responsible both for growing the plants used in their range of medicines and production.[2] A range of over-the-counter (OTC) products is available as tablets, powders, pilules, creams and lotions. Mother tinctures may occasionally be used. Many of the remedies can be prescribed on FP10 and are available on the National Health Service. Individualized medicines may be made to order from the vast array of mother tinctures stored by the manufacturer.

It is interesting to note that Boots has entered the market with its own range of homoeopathic medicines. The market opportunities are vast, when one considers that the current UK OTC market for homoeopathic medicines is about £12–16 million. In comparison, the market in France is £230 million and in Germany £210 million.[4]

References and further reading

1. Cook T. *Homoeopathic Medicine Today. A Modern Course of Study.* New Canaan: Keats, 1989.
2. Weleda – Information Video. Weleda UK, Ilkeston, Derbyshire.
3. Dellamour F, Brittan J. Importance of the 3C trituration in the manufacture of homoeopathic medicines. *Br Hom J* 1994; **83**: 8–14.
4. Lockie A. The over the counter market for homoeopathy. *Br Hom J* 1992; **81**: 199–200.
5. Gibson D. *Studies of Homoeopathic Remedies*. Beaconsfield: Beaconsfield Publishers, 1987.

4
The Organon

This book will not be devoted to the different views on homoeopathic philosophy; however in this chapter the importance of the *Organon* in homoeopathic thought will be considered. A later chapter will deal the views of other homoeopaths and their contributions to the present understanding of homoeopathy.

The *Organon* is a fascinating historical document charting the evolution of the thoughts of Hahnemann on the nature of the therapy he discovered. It was first published in 1810 in Coethen in Germany and ran to six editions. The final edition, with Hahnemann's hand-written alterations, is now in the possession of the University of California, San Francisco.[1]

The final (sixth) edition, written in 1842 shortly before Hahnemann's death, was not published until 1921, when it was rediscovered by Boericke and Haehl. Some radical changes to Hahnemann's previous views, such as LM (the fifty millesimal scale) potencies, contained in this document had been suppressed for nearly 80 years. During that time homoeopathic philosophy had taken different approaches; the Kentian school in the USA contrasted with the approach of Hughes in the UK.

The reason for the delay in publication is that Melanie, Hahnemann's second wife, is believed to have wanted the best possible price for the manuscript and persistently refused offers from homoeopaths from around the world to publish. After her death it was 'lost' until rediscovered in 1921. One can only speculate on the impact the sixth edition may have had on prominent contemporary homoeopaths such as James Tyler Kent, who never saw the document, as he died in 1918.

The *Organon* is presented as a series of aphorisms, 291 in all, and deserves repeated reading. It demonstrates Hahnemann's considerable understanding of the nature of disease, the homoeopathic principle, and the treatment of the individual. Although it would be difficult to cover all the document, it is worthwhile commenting on some of the leading aphorisms.

Aphorism	**Summary**
1	Defines the role of the physician in healing the sick.

2 The goal of therapy is to restore health rapidly, gently and permanently.

3 To achieve this using homoeopathy the physician must understand the nature of the disease, the medicine to be used, and then apply the medicine according to strict laws.

Each of the three principles described in aphorism 3 is discussed in detail later – the nature of disease in aphorisms 83–98, knowledge of the particular medicine in aphorisms 105–147 and the rules of use of medicine in aphorisms 150–280.

5 Hahnemann mentions the word ‘constitution’ as a factor in assessing the individual.

7 The *totality of symptoms*, defined as ‘the outer image expressing the inner essence of the disease’, is discussed, and its importance to correct remedy selection is stressed.

9 The vital force, a spirit-like dynamic force that animates the organism, is defined.

11 Illness is defined as the dynamic force being ‘untuned’.

12 ‘*It is only a pathologically untuned vital force that causes diseases*’.

17 *Cure* is defined as the *elimination of all perceptible signs and symptoms of the disease*. Hahnemann acknowledges the power of the mind to cause ill health.

18 The totality of symptoms and circumstances observed in each individual is the one and only guide to a choice of remedy.

22 To cure a disease a medicine must remove the subjective and objective symptoms of that disease. A *medicine* must produce artificial disease conditions similar to the disease in question. The medicine which is nearest to the totality of symptoms is most likely to cure.

24 The medicine produces an *artificial disease condition*, most likely to cure.

26 *In a living organism a weaker dynamic affection is extinguished by a stronger one*. The curative properties of a drug depend on its ability to resemble the disease, but act more strongly than it, and thus extinguish it.

34 Artificial disease caused by a medicine must not only be stronger than the disease, but also have the greatest possible similarity to it.

48 Only a medicine that produces similar symptoms to, and is stronger than, the disease can cure it.

52 This castigates the alternate use of allopathic and homoeopathic medicines.

58 This denigrates prescribing based on one or a few symptoms.

63 The mechanism of action of medicine is discussed – the *primary action*, followed by the *secondary action*. The stimulation of the vital force by a medicine is followed by a secondary action to preserve or restore the well-being of the organism.

72–80 Here Hahnemann discusses the origin of disease, both acute and chronic. He discusses the miasmatic nature of illness, but also identifies the role that psychological trauma can play in illness. He clearly predicts the nature of transmissible disease, and the influence of poor social conditions.

83–103 Hahnemann beautifully describes how to take an accurate homoeopathic history, including how to take into account other factors such as character and temperament when assessing the value of symptoms in the history (96).

108–147 Hahnemann describes the provings carried out on volunteers and gives precise instruction on the recording of data and interpreting symptoms.

150 An important comment: 'if someone complains of trifling symptoms of recent origin the physician should not consider it a fully fledged condition requiring serious medical attention' – a phrase many GPs would concur with today.

153 The importance of the *striking, strange, unusual* and *peculiar* symptom is discussed in the selection process when choosing a remedy.

156–158 *Aggravation*, the production of symptoms similar to the disease being treated, is discussed and the nature of the reaction explained: an aggravation is a highly similar medicinal disease which is stronger than the original complaint.

169 This discusses the importance of re-evaluating a case if an indicated remedy fails to act. One should not turn to a second-best choice, as the disease picture may have changed after administration of the first remedy.

174 *Local diseases*: this refers to external disease with few symptoms.

181 This discusses the use of a second remedy after a first remedy has produced an action.

186 Further definition of *local disease*. This stresses that inner problems are the cause of outer symptoms and signs.

195 The use of *antipsoric* remedies to cure residual complaints.

196–198 Decries the use of external medication to cure local external symptoms without treating the internal miasmatic disorder.

201 If a chronic disease cannot be overcome by the body, it forms a local disease externally to allay the internal disease.

204	The nature of chronic disease, predominantly *psora*, occasionally *psychosis* or *syphilis*.
208	Due regard must be given to social circumstances when assessing care.
210	*Psora*, a group of conditions predominantly affected by emotional and mental diseases. Stresses the importance of *mentals* in assessing a case.
211–230	Discusses the treatment of mental symptoms.
232	Alternating disease. The treatment of intermittent fevers.
246	Discusses the use of remedies, the dosage and repetition of the dose.
247	A *single dose* only should be given, and the result observed before repetition of dose.
252–253	The notion that there are obstacles to the curative action of the drug. The sign that a remedy is working is the psychic condition is improving, i.e. the mental symptoms are showing improvement.
260	Obstacles to cure are defined. As well as physical substances, the effects of grief, anger and mental strain are considered.
267	The preparation of the medicines is discussed.
269	Dynamization or potentiation is defined as the development of medicinal power.
270	The preparation and use of LM potencies and the use of 100 succussions is introduced as a new idea in the sixth edition (dilution 1 : 50 000).
273	Hahnemann discusses the use of the *single remedy*, at one time, and not repeated until the action of the medicine is exhausted.
276	The effect of an incorrect dose or potency of remedy is discussed.
280	Repetition of the dose in increasing strength is allowed when one or more of the old or original symptoms reappears.
282	Homoeopathic aggravation: '*a heightening of the original disease symptoms observed...then this is a sure sign that the doses were too large*'.
286–290	The effect of mesmerism is discussed by Hahnemann.

Why produce this list of aphorisms? I noted over the years that when there were problems understanding the philosophy and practice of homoeopathy I frequently had to refer to the *Organon*. Understanding and rereading these aphorisms in the context of how you practise can be very rewarding. I believe those I have emphasized in *italic* type are the most important. In a later chapter I will discuss the influence of other homoeopathic philosophers on modern thought.

References and further reading

1. Schmidt J. History and relevance of the 6th edition of the Organon of medicine (1842). *Br Hom J* 1994; **83**: 42–48.
2. Hahnemann S. *Organon of Medicine.* (Translated by Kunzli J, Naude A, Pendleton P.) London: Victor Gollancz, 1992.
3. Clover A. Back to basics (George McLeod lecture). *Br Hom J* 1996; **85**: 75–78.

5

The Chronic Diseases

Hahnemann's three major works are the *Organon, Materia Medica Pura* and his later writings on the chronic diseases, entitled *The Chronic Diseases. Their Peculiar Nature and their Homoeopathic Cure*. This last text was first published in 1828, a time when many observers felt that Hahnemann was already in intellectual decline. It ran to five volumes, the last being published in 1838.

The book appears to have been written as a summary of Hahnemann's experiences over many years treating various conditions which did not completely respond to acute treatment, and would reappear.

Hahnemann postulated that there was some fundamental underlying reason for the recurrence of these illnesses. He believed that the acute problems were part of a deeper, more complex illness.

The philosophy of the *Chronic Diseases* is much debated. One reason is that some newer antipsoric medicines used to treat chronic illnesses were proven on sick people, rather than in healthy volunteers, as demanded so strictly in the *Organon*.

Hahnemann based his explanation of the chronic illnesses on his *theory of miasm*. Miasm is defined as 'polluting exhalations, or malarial poisons' and perhaps a more appropriate term would have been stigmata. Hahnemann believed that all miasms were passed from generation to generation, and he believed that medicines only suppressed, but did not cure, the miasm.

He believed that all chronic disease is a result of particular diseases which are already known. He referred to those conditions due to suppressed skin eruptions, particularly scabies, as *psora*. This is the most prevalent of the chronic diseases. For this he made a remedy from the scabies vesicle. This was the first nosode.

The psoric miasm is the most common miasm and must exist before the other miasms; it exhibits a variety of symptoms. Patients are chilly and lack vital heat. Their mental symptoms include introversion, anxiety and anticipatory worries. They are hesitant and slow thinkers. They are best in the morning. They suffer from skin problems and degenerative disorders.

The *sycotic* miasm is related to gonorrhoea, and the *syphilitic* miasm to syphilis. Other miasms were thought by Hahnemann to arise from combinations of the above.

The *tubercular* miasm is a combination of either sycotic or syphilitic miasm with the psoric miasm, and the *cancerous* miasm is a combination of all three.

Hahnemann used his miasmatic theory to analyse cases where the 'best indicated remedy' failed to act. He assessed which miasm was dominant and gave the appropriate remedy.

The place of miasmatic theory in homoeopathy depends on the practitioner. I have met many homoeopaths who always prescribe miasmatically if possible. Equally, I have met many successful doctors who rarely use this approach. In the future this is an area that will need further exploration.

Further reading

1. Speight P. *A Comparison of Chronic Miasms*. Bradford Holdsworthy: Devon Homoeopathic Group, 1992.
2. Bannerjee PK. *Chronic Disease. Its Cause and Cure*. New Delhi: B Jain Publishers, 1988 (reprint).
3. Robert H. *The Principles and Art of Cure by Homoeopathy*. New Delhi: B Jain Publishers, 1988 (reprint). 1979.

6

The scientific investigation of homoeopathy

(It all sounds very interesting, but where's the proof?)

This is a common quote from sceptics who do not believe in the value of homoeopathy. However I do believe that there is a growing body of evidence in the form of both randomized studies and anecdotal information, of the benefits of homoeopathy.

Recent consumer surveys show that the public is not deterred by the reluctance of the health care professions to adopt complementary medicines. In 1993 the *Daily Telegraph* sampled a large population and found that 96% had used a form of alternative medicine. Some 77% of respondents had found the therapy useful and 94% would consider using them again.[1]

In 1993 the National Association of Health Authorities and Trusts published the findings of a survey into the use of complementary therapies within the National Health Service (NHS). They looked particularly at purchasers' attitudes to the availability of therapies within the NHS.

More than 70% of Family Health Service Authorities (FHSAs) and GP fundholders and 65% of District Health Authorities (DHAs) were in favour of some therapies being available on the NHS. A total of 60% of DHAs, 65% of FHSAs and 50% of GP fundholders thought homoeopathy should be available. This surely demonstrates a groundswell of support for its use.[2]

A survey by the Consumers' Association in 1986 reported that about 12% of their readers had used some form of alternative therapy in the previous 12 months. Again, over 80% noted some improvement on the therapies, and three-quarters would use the therapies again. The most popular therapies were osteopathy (42%), homoeopathy (28%), acupuncture (23%), chiropractic (22%) and herbalism (11%).[3]

However the era of evidence-based medicine is also upon us, and it behoves those working in homoeopathy to demonstrate the efficacy of the therapy when competing for scarce resources. Homoeopathy cannot rely on anecdote alone. If it is to maintain the momentum achieved over recent years then scientific investigation must be encouraged.

Evidence-based medicine, although in vogue, has come in for criticism from eminent health experts for meeting the needs of populations, but not the needs of the individual.[4]

Many purists believe this is folly, as the use of a remedy is based on the individuality of the patient. However, as I will discuss, attempts have been made to show the benefits of homoeopathy even using this allopathic method of scientific evaluation. Whilst many may argue that allopathic medicine has itself not been fully evaluated, and that perhaps only 15–20% of what we practise conventionally is based on sound science,[5] it is still the responsibility of those working in the field to try and demonstrate the benefits.

However anecdote should not be devalued: McNaughton states: 'Anecdotes and stories, therefore, are integral to medical practice and to the education of those practising it. Learning the scientific basis for understanding people is only one part of the holistic approach to which students must aspire'.[6]

Other physicians understand the need to view science with a certain degree of scepticism. It is estimated by some that 1 in 20 hospital admissions are due to a drug given by their physician.

The scientific study of homoeopathy

Homoeopathy has never been able to attract the massive funding available to other disciplines. A system of medicine that is outside the mainstream and which by its very nature suggests that there is another way of treating people than the use of drugs will certainly not attract the funding given to conventional doctors for research purposes. Over the decades homoeopathic doctors have attempted to study the homoeopathic effect scientifically. More recently researchers in physics and molecular biology have begun to investigate the mechanism by which homoeopathy works.

Therapeutic effect

If homoeopathic medicine is a placebo then it has stood the test of time. Placebo effects are supposed to occur in up to 40% of individuals who take an inactive substance. And yet results better than placebo have been demonstrated with homoeopathic preparations using good scientific methodology.

Much of the work of the general practitioner – kindness, empathy and reassurance – could be perceived as placebo effect, where the patient's condition seems to change due to the act of receiving treatment rather than the treatment itself.[7]

If the homoeopathic effect is purely placebo, then the question has to be asked: why do infants respond so well? Why do animals who have had their water troughs dosed significantly improve when given homoeopathy? It is the task of researchers to prove that the method is effective when judged by modern scientific methods.

In 1941 Paterson and Boyd looked at whether high potencies were clinically active. They examined a comparison of a potentized dose of diphtherinum and alum-precipitated toxoid and observed reduced susceptibility to diphtheria using the Schick test in the potentized group.[8]

In 1943[9] tests on potentized mustard gas were designed to see if they were able to modify skin lesions produced by application of the gas to the skin. Results suggested the remedies used were statistically superior to placebo. They reduced the severity of the burn, and Rhus tox. prevented excessive sensitization to those exposed to a skin application of mustard gas.

Over the years there have been numerous case reports of the remarkable successes of homoeopathy. In 1987 Beneveniste[10] appeared to have made a breakthrough in explaining the mechanism of action of homoeopathy. It has been postulated that during the preparation of a homoeopathic remedy the process of succussion somehow implants on the molecule of water a ‘message’. The water molecule retains the memory and it is this that is its therapeutic action. Beneveniste, in his experiments using potentized immunoglobulin E, claimed that in a highly diluted solution with no active ingredient he was still able to demonstrate mast cell degranulation as evidence of activity of the potentized solution. This was published in *Nature*, and subsequently the method was scrutinized and criticized. An investigative team was sent to his laboratories but was unable to reproduce the evidence using similar methods.

In 1986 Brigo and colleagues in Italy assessed the effect of homoeopathy on recurrent migraine. Using a variety of selected remedies a significant reduction in the intensity and frequency of migraine was noted.[11]

Taylor-Reilly in 1986 produced a paper demonstrating the homoeopathic effect which was not due to placebo. This double-blind randomized trial using mixed-grass pollen on patients suffering from seasonal rhinitis displayed a clear reduction in symptoms and antihistamine usage.[12]

Fisher in 1989 studied the effects of rhus tox. 6C on patients suffering from primary fibromyalgia. Using double-blind techniques, clear evidence emerged of a therapeutic effect.

In 1994 Reilly published a paper in the *Lancet*, 'Is evidence for homoeopathy reproducible?', which demonstrated in a trial of 24 patients with allergic asthma that significant and prolonged improvement occurred compared with placebo, using allergen material.[13]

A meta-analysis of 122 trials of homoeopathy carried out by Dutch observers concluded that, although many of the studies looked at were flawed in their design, overall there was convincing evidence for the need to continue research as benefit appeared to be obtained.[14]

If the above suggests that homoeopathy does work, then an explanation of how it works is also needed. Reading the *British Homoeopathic Journal* it is clear that there are many molecular biologists, physicists and philosophers working in this field.

The homoeopathic effect – scientific models

Rubik, in an excellent review,[15] describes the dilemmas facing those trying to enhance the reputation of homoeopathy, and discusses the resistance scientists meet in acknowledging data that contradict their own hypothesis. The problems faced by researchers in this field include factors such as difficulty in publishing, difficulty in funding, obstacles to promotion when proposing alternative models, loss of employment, and the critical backlash which inevitably follows. She concludes that conventional science maintains that biological functions are still retained by the DNA, and ignores the possibility of theories such as 'water memory', and that low-level non-ionizing electromagnetic fields can produce biological effects.

Scientific models for the action of homoeopathy abound. Fundamental to the credible explanations is the effect of potentization on the water molecule. Biophysical models are being investigated worldwide using the assumption that energy fields of a physically measurable nature are the explanation for the medicine's effect.

The methods of preparation of the homoeopathic substance – succussion and serial dilution – are more important to the process of understanding the theory of action of the medicines. The theories suggest that potentized water solutions consist of water molecules bound together via hydrogen bonds in an organized manner, but the three-dimensional structure alters with the presence of solutes.

It is stated that spectrographic analysis of potentized medicines shows that they differ in their infrared absorption patterns at the frequency associated with hydroxy bonds. Further, the crystallization patterns of ice differs, depending on the potency of the solution. Thus it is possible that there may be a change in the crystalline structure of water molecules and their ability to absorb and emit radiation at specific frequencies.[16] How would water store the information of energized potencies?

Some feel that specific isotopes in a crystal network store information. Armed with this theory, one still needs to understand how this can possibly work at the therapeutic level. Using the models discussed, Towsey and Hasan[16] tried to deduce a mechanism by which homoeopathy acts. They believe that the crystalline structure of water is altered by the molecules that imprint the 'message' during succussion. As the molecules disappear during serial dilution, they postulate that the already altered crystal structure somehow multiplies and produces more altered forms of the energized water molecule, each with similar vibrational characteristics.

The potentized liquids emit radiation at a specific frequency which has a physiological effect upon enzyme activity. The authors conclude that homoeopathic medicines act by biophysical and not biochemical methods.[16]

Another interesting viewpoint is the application of Sheldrake's theories on morphic resonance to the model of homoeopathic action.[17] Those fields of energy which surround all living systems can transmit their energy field even during potentization and somehow be stored in what is described by Vithoulkas and Anagnostatos[17] as a 'clathrate mantle' – a form of storage of information in the solution in which potentization is taking place.[16]

Theoretical models for the homoeopathic effect abound. Poitevin[18] suggests that the scientific principles of homoeopathy do not require a new paradigm, but could be incorporated into those currently known biological regulatory processes which are, as yet, imperfectly understood.

Modern homoeopathic thought

In the latter part of the 19th century the 'schism' that divided homoeopaths addressed the issue of potency. The Kentian school advocated high-potency constitutional prescribing, whilst the followers of Hughes advocated low-potency pathological prescribing. The Kentian school prevailed and in the UK homoeopathy has kept to the classical approach. Other countries, such as France and Germany, have adapted and experimented. The Germans in particular use complex homoeopathic preparations and the French are innovative in their approaches using multiple therapy (pluralism), organotherapy and gemmotherapy.[19]

One of the most prominent contemporary homoeopaths is George Vithoulkas, an experienced non-medically qualified homoeopath whose views on homoeopathy, health and the role of allopathic medicine are challenging, to say the least. In his latest book,[20] Vithoulkas attacks the failures of conventional medicine and blames their side-effects for many of the illnesses the world is currently experiencing. His theory is that our immune systems are unable to deal with new diseases as a result of the chronic overuse of antibiotics.

Vithoulkas proposes a new model of how health is maintained on three planes – the mental–spiritual, the emotional–psychic and the physical–material. Using these planes as his new model for health he describes in detail how disorders such as acquired immunodeficiency syndrome (AIDS) have arisen and how using only the energized medicines of homoeopathy human beings can recover the ability to heal themselves.

Homoeopathy and the holistic view

A number of factors helped shape the current view of modern bio-medicine.The 18th and 19th centuries saw the development of the modern sciences of anatomy, physiology and bacteriology; there were also significant advances in pharmacology and diagnostic technologies in this century. A mechanistic view of illness evolved. Philosophers such as René Descartes, in his book *Treatise on Man*, distinguished the spiritual world from the material world. He likened everything within that world, including the human body, to a machine. The machine could be analysed by examining function and form. In modern-technology medicine this has led to the separation of body and mind, with the focus on their individual parts. Along with changes in the provision of health care in the 18th century, a *positivist* approach to health care developed. According to positivism, all things around us can be observed, measured and relationships identified between those things measured and observed. This cause-and-effect relationship can then be translated into hypotheses and theories about the nature of ill health.

Homoeopathy, like many complementary therapies, as they are now called, takes a holistic view. Holism tends to emphasize the fundamental wholeness of the human being and the therapies stress the importance of balance within the organism. Following from this, it is recognized that disease is a result of an imbalance in the individual. Holism recognizes the importance of environmental, psychological and social factors in the development of disease and as an aid to recovery.

An important feature of all complementary therapies is that they recognize the potential of the body to heal itself, as well as individuals taking responsibility for their own health. It will be seen later in this book that many of these concepts are recognized as integral to the homoeopathic approach.

The holistic view is being adopted by many more conventionally trained practitioners. My own experience in training general practitioners and nurses is that there is an increasing awareness of the limitations of conventional medicine. Their training is beginning to embrace issues which address the importance of the practitioner–patient relationship, counselling, and patients taking increasing responsibility for their health and well-being, both physically and mentally. The holistic model has been adopted by many in the primary care setting, and one of the beauties of primary care is that it adapts and incorporates changes in practice for the benefit of the patients. The range of complementary services now on offer in many practices is testament to this.

Criticism of homoeopathy

Homoeopathy has many detractors and it would be naive to ignore their criticisms. One of the most damning books about complementary therapy is that by Skrabanek and McCormick,[22] who believe that the debate about the efficacy of homoeopathy ended with the failed Beneveniste experiments. It is an entertaining read as it also finds little to praise in many of the methods used in conventional medicine. What the book fails to answer is why so many people still turn to these therapies and what is lacking in conventional medicine that makes them feel the need to do so. They believe that all complementary therapies are placebos and that their effect is often due to the enthusiasm of the practitioner, but do not explain some of the dramatic improvements made by patients and why there have been positive double-blind studies reported, such as those of Taylor-Reilly.[12, 13] The debate continues!

References and further reading

1. Doyle C. Reaching out for an alternative. *Daily Telegraph* 1993.
2. NAHAT. *Complementary Therapies in the NHS.* Research paper no. 10. London: NAHAT, 1993.
3. Magic or medicine? *Which*? 1996; October 443–447.
4. The NHS handbook criticises evidence based medicine. *Br Med J* 1996; **312**: 1439.
5. Quality control for medicine. *New Sci* 1994; **143**. (1943): 22–24.
6. McNaughton J. Anecdotes and empiricism. *Br J Gen Pract* 1995; **45**: 571–572.
7. What difference do GPs make? *BMA News Rev* 1994 (December): 12–14.
8. Paterson J, Boyd, W.E. Potency action: a preliminary study of the alteration of the Schick test by a homoeopathic potency. *Br Hom J* 1941; **31**: No. 5.
9. Report by the special committee of the British Homoeopathic Society to the Ministry of Home Security on Mustard Gas experiments. *Br Hom J* 1943; **33**(2).

10. Davenas E, Beaurais F, Amara J *et al.* Human basophil degranulation triggered by very dilute anti-serum against IgE. *Nature* 1988; **333**: 816–818.
11. Brigo B, Serpellari G, *et al.* Homoeopathic treatment of migraine: randomised double blind controlled study of 60 cases. *Berlin J Res Homoeopathy* 1991; **1**: 98–106.
12. Reilly D. Is homoeopathy a placebo response? Controlled trial of homoeopathic potency with pollen in hayfever. *Lancet* 1986; **ii**: 881–886.
13. Reilly D. Is the evidence for homoeopathy reproducible? *Lancet* 1994; **344**: 1601–1606.
14. Kleijnen J, Knipschild P, ter Riet G. Clinical trials of homoeopathy. *Br Med J* 1991; **302**: 316–323.
15. Rubik B. The perennial challenge of anomalies at the frontiers of science. *Br Hom J*.1994; **83**: 155–166.
16. Towsey M, Hasan MY. Homoeopathy – a biophysical point of view. *Br Hom J* 1995; **84**.
17. Van Galen E. Homoeopathy and morphic resonance. *Br Hom J* 1994; **83**.
18. Poitevin B. Mechanism of action of homoeopathic medicines. *Br Hom J* 1995; **84**: 32–39.
19. Eizagaya F. The international homoeopathic movement. *Br Hom J* **84**: 1995; 67–70.
20. Vithoulkas G. *A New Model of Health and Disease*. Berkeley, CA: North Atlantic Books, 1991.
21. Aggleton P. *Health*. London: Routledge; 1993.
22. Skrabanek P, McCormick J. *Follies and Fallacies in Medicine*. Chippenham: Tarragon Press, 1994 (reprint).

7

The development of homoeopathy in the UK

There is evidence to suggest that homoeopathy was being used, albeit temporarily, before 1831 by some of the nobility. However it is recognized that the person responsible for establishing the reputation of homoeopathy was Frederick Foster Hervey Quin, who settled in London in 1832. Quin was a remarkable person with a colourful past. He was thought to be the illegitimate son of the Duchess of Devonshire, and enjoyed her considerable patronage.

In 1818 at the age of 19 he obtained his MD from Edinburgh University after only 3 years. His first employment was as physician to the exiled Napoleon Bonaparte on the island of St Helena; however, Napoleon died before Quin was able to take up his appointment. Quin therefore travelled with the Duchess of Devonshire as her personal physician on a tour of Europe. Quin was taken seriously ill in Italy, and was cared for by the famous Italian homoeopath Dr Romani.

In 1842, following the death of his patron, Quin decided to study homoeopathy. He learnt German and translated the *Organon* into English. He studied with Romani, before eventually travelling to Germany to learn from the master himself – Hahnemann. Whilst in Germany he met Prince Leopold, Queen Victoria's uncle, who was later to become a patron. For 3 years Quin practised in Paris, until his return to London in 1832.

Quin's charm and personality won him many devotees. His contacts with the aristocracy ensured a thriving practice and a growth of interest in homoeopathy.

In 1843 a homoeopathic society was founded by Quin and his contemporaries. This was to become the forerunner of the Faculty of Homoeopathy, founded in 1943.

In 1850 the first homoeopathic hospital opened in Golden Square, London, before the terrible cholera epidemic of 1854. An analysis of the outcome of treatments for cholera showed that the mortality rates of patients at all hospitals was 53.2%, compared to only 16.4% at the homoeopathic hospital.

A bill drawn up by Parliament to forbid any practice of medicine other than that taught by medical colleges attempted to outlaw the practice of homoeopathy. It was only due to the diligence of Lord Ebury, a supporter of Quin's, who reminded the House of the success of homoeopathy against cholera, that the bill was not passed.

These figures were reviewed by a House of Lords committee, which gave recognition to the use of homoeopathy as a therapy and allayed much of the prejudice propounded by allopathic doctors at a time when some conventional doctors were attempting to have its practice banned.

In 1878 Quin died, bequeathing £10 000 to the London Homoeopathic Hospital.

Other prominent homoeopaths

Richard Hughes is another famous name in the history of homoeopathy. He and Dr JH Clarke dominated British homoeopathy at the turn of this century. Hughes is famous for his views that homoeopathy could be practised using low-potency remedies based on the patient's pathological picture, placing less emphasis on the mental and general symptom picture.

These views developed into the schism that was to divide the homoeopathic profession, and he and Clarke became bitter opponents.

Hughes was a prodigious writer. The most famous of his publications are *A Manual of Pharmacodynamics, The Principles and Practice of Homoeopath*, and the *Cyclopaedia of Drug Pathogenesis*.

Hughes used low-potency medicines, although he acknowledged the success of potencies used by colleagues up to 200C, and he was not convinced by the American school of thought using the higher potencies.

Hughes dominated the homoeopathic scene until his death in Dublin in 1902. Over the ensuing years there was a backlash against his teaching. Many British homoeopaths adopted the Kentian school of thinking – high-potency, constitutional prescribing. This was partly because its advocates John Weir and Margaret Tyler had the opportunity to travel and study with Kent thanks to a scholarship donated by Dr Tyler.

Although Hughes is out of favour as a half-homoeopath, I am sure many doctors today are currently prescribing using the pathological low-dose approach, with much success.

As noted previously, Sir John Weir was a convert to homoeopathy having come under the influence of the homoeopath Gibson-Miller. Weir travelled to the USA and studied at the Hering Homoeopathic College. On his return he became an advocate of Kent's and promoted his teachings in the UK. With the help of Margaret Tyler and others, Weir began the radical promotion of homoeopathy. In 1911 he was appointed Professor of Materia Medica and he began a regular education programme of meetings and courses.

In 1932 he was invited to speak to the Royal Society of Medicine, an event which signalled a recognition of homoeopathy and the status of Weir himself as its advocate.

Weir was appointed royal physician to King George V and was knighted in 1932. His contribution was the introduction of an educational programme and the promotion of the Kentian school of thought in the UK.

He died in 1971, and was succeeded by Dr Marjorie Blackie. Dr Blackie is responsible for the revival of interest in recent years amongst doctors. She developed a short course in homoeopathy and promoted the MFHom examination.

Marjorie Blackie joined the staff of the London Homoeopathic Hospital in 1924, and was influenced by the teachings of Clarke, Wheeler and Borland; Borland was a former pupil of James Tyler Kent in the USA. Blackie ran a busy homoeopathic general practice alongside her hospital work. She was Dean of the Faculty of Homoeopathy from 1965 to 1979.

Blackie was an advocate of the use of high-potency 10M prescribing for constitutional cases, and 6C potency for local cases. Her works include *Classical Homoeopathy* and *The Patient not the Cure*.

The recent research work of Dr David Reilly at Glasgow Homoeopathic Hospital and Dr Peter Fisher at the Royal London Homoeopathic Hospital, amongst others, has done much to enhance the scientific credibility of homoeopathy, an area much criticized by our allopathic colleagues. Their work is discussed in Chapter 6.

Homoeopathy is enjoying a growth in interest amongst medical practitioners. Currently courses are held at Bristol, Liverpool, Glasgow and the Royal London Homoeopathic Hospitals. There are currently 220 fellows and members and 800 associates of the Faculty.

The recent introduction of the primary care certificate should ensure a growing demand for educational facilities for GPs and primary care workers wanting to learn more.[1]

Homoeopathic hospitals

Homoeopathy was incorporated into the National Health Service (NHS) in 1948. Several institutions developed during the latter part of the 19th century to provide homoeopathic services. Today there are five prominent centres: London, Glasgow, Liverpool, Bristol and Tunbridge Wells. As a result of the introduction of fundholding and the increased demand for homoeopathic services, there has been an increase in the number of outpatient clinics in areas such as Sidmouth, Dalkeith and Powys, as well as practice-based clinics.

London

As mentioned previously, the first London hospital opened in 1850 at Golden Square, London. This moved to Great Ormond Street in 1859, with further extensions in 1893.

In 1937 the hospital achieved royal patronage on the coronation of George VI. In 1948 it was renamed the Royal London Homoeopathic Hospital. It retains the premier status of the main teaching institution for homoeopathy in the UK and its reputation is acknowledged around the world. The recent changes in the NHS and the new model purchaser–provider split enabled the hospital to become an independent trust, promoting its services to a wider area, and fostering development of an increased range of services, including a variety of complementary therapies, outpatient and inpatient services and teaching facilities.

Glasgow

Glasgow had its first homoeopathic dispensary in 1880. A new unit was opened in 1909 under the guidance of its first physician, Dr Gibson-Miller. The present hospital in Great Western Road is a recognized centre for teaching and research under the guidance of Dr David Reilly, whose work on establishing scientific method and well-conducted scientific trials has done much to enhance the credibility of homoeopathy. Glasgow pioneered the Primary Care Certificate in Homoeopathy, which is now a recognized qualification by the Faculty for beginners. Glasgow is currently planning to build a new hospital to expand its range of services. Approximately 15% of Scottish GPs have some training in homoeopathy and the Primary Health Care Certificate is likely to promote an increase in these numbers.[1]

Liverpool

A homoeopathic dispensary was founded in Liverpool in 1842. In 1849, after a cholera epidemic in which homoeopathic treatment was particularly successful, a benefactor in the form of the Tate family built and equipped the Liverpool Hahnemann Hospital. Until recently the hospital was based at Mosseley Hill Hospital until its closure, with the loss of inpatient beds. Currently outpatients are still seen at Mosseley Hill under the supervision of a consultant in homoeopathic medicine.

Bristol

The Bristol Hospital at Cotham Hill was built following a gift from the Wills (tobacco) family. It was opened in 1925 and replaced a smaller hospital in the city.

Sadly, Bristol lost its grand inpatient hospital facilities in 1992. However a new purpose-built outpatient department was recently opened and it is thriving with Dr David Spence as medical director.

Tunbridge Wells

The hospital began as a dispensary in 1863. It moved to larger premises in 1887 and opened as a hospital in 1890. The hospital still has a consultant supervising the care of patients, as well as a thriving outpatient department.

Homoeopathy and royal patronage

It has been to the benefit of homoeopathy that it has enjoyed royal patronage both in the UK and abroad. This initially stems from Hahnemann's contacts with the various royal houses of Germany. Many of the nobles treated by Hahnemann were relatives of Queen Victoria. Hahnemann's benefactor at one time was the father of Prince Albert, who later married Queen Victoria.

The first patron was Queen Adelaide, wife of William IV; she was a German princess who had used homoeopathy all her life. King George V used homoeopathy extensively, and appointed the first royal homoeopathic physician.

King George VI, father of our present monarch, also used homoeopathy, and even named one of his race horses after a remedy. This horse, Hypericum, won the 2000 guineas in 1949.

Today members of the present royal family still use homoeopathy.

Homoeopathy in the NHS

It has perhaps ironic that homoeopathy, though still vilified by many doctors and scientists, was at one time the only form of complementary medicine available within the NHS. This was as a result of the incorporation of all hospitals into the scheme in 1948, which allowed the use of homoeopathy to continue; however, there have been many attempts over the decades to encourage its demise despite the increasing demand from patients. Swayne estimates that there may be at least

750 000 consultations taking place each year in the NHS, but this is probably a gross underestimate because of lack of accurate data.[2]

Homoeopathy abroad

USA and Latin America

Although several notable doctors practised in the USA in the early years of the 19th century, perhaps the greatest was Constantine Hering. He was initially a sceptic: whilst still an undergraduate at Leipzig University he was asked to write an essay on the dubious practice of homoeopathy by his teacher Dr Robbi. His research, however, led him to embrace the discipline, and when he moved to the USA in 1833, he began practising there. In 1844 he helped set up the American Institute of Homoeopathy.

As a result of this, American allopathic doctors felt threatened. They founded the American Medical Association (AMA) and over the next 60 years began a concerted campaign to ostracize homoeopaths.

The other great name in homoeopathy in the USA is James Tyler Kent (1849–1916), whose works include the *Repertory, Lectures in Homoeopathic Philosophy* and *The Materia Medica*. It was Kent who returned to the practice of strict Hahnemannian principles, using the single dose, advocating the use of high potencies, and no repetition of the dose if improvement was being maintained. His teachings were adopted by many of the foremost British homoeopaths of this century.

The continued antagonism of the AMA and the rise of modern western medicine, including anaesthetics and antibiotics, saw the decline in popularity of homoeopathy in the 1920s. In more recent years, despite homoeopathy being banned in certain states, there has been a revival in interest in its practice.[3] Several colleges promote its use and are involved in training. Complementary medicine is enjoying a boom in the USA, with an estimated $13.7 billion dollars spent in 1993. The number of consultations with alternative practitioners exceeds the number of consultations with primary care physicians. Forty medical schools include teaching on alternative medicine in their curriculum.[4]

In Latin America, particularly Brazil, Argentina and Mexico, teaching is highly developed and there are an estimated 30 000 practitioners.

Europe

Homoeopathy is practised in many countries throughout Europe. There is a vast difference in how homoeopathy is viewed amongst the

European nations. In the UK it is legal and offered as part of the NHS; it was officially recognized in 1950 with the granting of a royal charter.

The Scandinavian countries recognize the therapy but restrict who can practise. In Belgium and Italy (and Jersey!) it lacks official recognition.

In France there are 25 000 physicians who prescribe homoeopathy. Germany has developed a 3-year training programme for those wishing to be called homoeopathic physicians. There is also a training programme for non-medically qualified homoeopaths called *Heilpraktiker*.

In Greece educational requirements are 6 years of homoeopathic practice. Homoeopathic medicines are prescription-only.

In Italy the nosodes are banned and practice is restricted.

In Spain the Spanish Medical Council supports homoeopathy practised by doctors only.[5] Non-medically qualified practitioners are banned in France and Belgium, but have unlimited freedom to practise in the UK, Holland and Denmark.

European homoeopaths are united via the European Committee for Homoeopathy, a legal body whose statutes are approved by the Belgian government. The aim of the body is to exchange information, develop relations between participants, set objectives and approve a budget.

The Liga Medicorum Homoeopatica Internationalis (LMHI) is a worldwide body linking homoeopaths and fostering links via an annual congress.[6]

India

In India, where homoeopathy is used extensively, homoeopaths may have been practising as early as 1810. Julian Hoenigberger recorded the practice of homoeopathy in India before 1852 and was himself trained by Hahnemann. He returned to India and was appointed as physician to the court of Lahore.

India is unique in its number of homoeopaths, both lay and medically qualified, and also because the practice of homoeopathy is endorsed by the government. In 1972 there were estimated to be 70 000 registered practitioners, and up to 300 000 practitioners in total. Currently the Indian Health Service is subdivided within the Ministry of Health into Modern Medicine and Homoeopathy and Alternative Systems of Medicine.[7]

References and further reading

1. Reilly D. A certificate of primary care homoeopathy. *Br Hom J* 1994; **83**: 57–58.

2. Swayne J. Survey of the use of homoeopathic medicine in the UK health system. *J R Coll Gen Pract* 1989; **39**: 503–506.
3. Editorial. Homoeopathy banned in US state. *Br Hom J* 1990; **81**: 1–2.
4. International round up of alternative medicine. *Br Med J* 1996; **313**.
5. Segall E. Landmark meeting of the European Committee for Homoeopathy. *Homoeopathy* 1996; **46**: (3): 14–16.
6. Summary of the 50th Congress of LHMI. *Homoeopathy* March 1996.
7. Ruthren-Mitchell. *Homoeopathy*. London: WH Allen, 1975.

8

Comparison of related therapies

It may seem inappropriate to discuss other forms of therapy in a book about homoeopathy. However, one of the most frustrating aspects of practising any form of complementary medicine is how patients group therapies into one, assuming they are all the same. This leads to confusion for the patient: the practitioner must have a basic understanding of other treatments so as to be able to explain the differences and similarities. I am in no way an expert on these therapies, but have found that those listed below are commonly confused with homoeopathy.

Anthroposophical medicine

This system of medicine was based on the teachings of Rudolph Steiner (1861–1925), an Austrian philosopher. The term derived from the Greek – *anthropos*, meaning human being, and *sophos*, meaning wise. Although not as popular in the UK as in Europe, it still enjoys a considerable following.

The remedies are not purely homoeopathic: some are diluted, others diluted and succussed. The remedies are used in such a way as to match the remedy with the affinity for a certain organ or system. Some of the remedies have not been proved. Some remedies are mixed together in different potencies. Anthroposophical medicine may use other approaches such as hydrotherapy and massage, art therapy and movement therapy, called therapeutic eurhythmy.

The anthroposophical model classified illnesses according to the particular systems affected. All three systems were related and interconnected – nerves and senses; metabolism and musculoskeletal system; and circulation and respiration.

As with many complementary therapies, there is an associated philosophy regarding lifestyle and the relationship between the physical body and the astral body.

Bach flower remedies

Dr Edward Bach, a homoeopathic physician who discovered with Paterson the bowel nosodes in the 1930s, developed a therapeutic system known as the flower remedies.

Bach believed that certain mental states predisposed the individual to ill health. These illnesses could be treated by taking the flower remedies.

The remedies were grouped according to the emotional state or type of personality. There are seven groups including fear, uncertainty, disinterest or apathy, loneliness, oversensitivity to external stimuli, despondency and despair, and excessive care for the welfare of others. The remedies differ in each group and within a group the severity of the condition may indicate a particular remedy.

The flower remedies are not produced in the same way as homoeopathic remedies. Many patients I see for homoeopathic treatment have used, or are using, flower remedies; particularly popular is the rescue remedy, a combination of five remedies used for emotional emergencies.

Biochemic remedies

The tissue salts or biochemic remedies were first described by Wilhelm Schuessler in 1873. A homoeopathic physician by training, Schuessler believed that illness occurred as a result of an imbalance of the mineral salts within the body. He named 12 salts that could be used singly or together to treat these conditions. The salts are prepared homoeopathically to a potency of 6C.

The salts include:

1. Calc. fluor.
2. Calc. phos.
3. Calc. sulph.
4. Ferr. phos.
5. Kali. mur.
6. Kali. phos.
7. Kali. sulp.
8. Mag. phos.
9. Nat. mur.
10. Nat. phos.
11. Nat. sulph.
12. Silica

Close examination of the symptom picture reveals similarities between these remedies used homoeopathically and as biochemic remedies, and also many differences.

The tissue salts can also be found as combination remedies to treat specific groups of conditions.

Complex homoeopathy

Complex homoeopathy was developed by Hahnemann's pupils. It involves the mixing of low-potency preparations (6C and 12C) and mother tinctures, and combines the effects of homoeopathy and herbalism. The herbal elements of the therapy concentrate on the beneficial drainage effects on a particular organ.

Complex homoeopathy is particularly well-developed in Germany, where about 80% of all homoeopathic remedies are in this form. It is believed by its practitioners that using the combinations of remedies is particularly well-suited to the management of chronic diseases.

Herbalism

The use of herbs to cure ill health has been practised for centuries. The Chinese have used herbs for thousands of years, and herbalism is one branch of traditional Chinese medicine.

Herbalism clearly differs from homoeopathy in that the latter uses dilute potentized medicines whereas the former uses material doses of the herbs required. This still causes confusion amongst patients, who believe that homoeopathy and herbalism are the same thing.

Herbalists and their remedies use the principle of 'simpling', where the whole plant is used to produce a medicine. It is argued that the natural balance within the plant is crucial for the therapeutic effect, rather than trying to isolate an active ingredient.

Herbal remedies can detoxify a system and eliminate waste, strengthen the organism and help in the healing process, and also strengthen specific organs.

Herbal remedies can be given as infusions, tinctures, poultices, liniments, syrups and salves. Oils can be used to make cream for massage.

Medical herbalists in the UK are highly trained practitioners who undergo a 4-year programme, which includes fundamental health sciences, clinical examination and therapeutics as well as teaching on the use of herbs.

Naturopathy

This system of therapeutics finds more favour in other European countries than in the UK. It is based on the principle that the vital force familiar to homoeopaths is disturbed by the accumulation of poisons within the body. Naturopaths take a view that preventive medicine through education is important. The naturopath aims to treat the complaint by eliminating the poisons and allowing the body to heal itself, with the minimum of outside interference.

Diet and fasting play an important part in the healing process. The naturopath may combine this with other treatments such as hydrotherapy, herbal medicine, osteopathy, homoeopathy, acupuncture or a variety of other therapies.

Further reading

1. Newman Turner R. *Naturopathic Medicine: Treating the Whole Person*, revised edn. Wellingborough:Thorsons, 1990.
2. Pahlow M. *Living Medicine: The Healing Properties of Plants*. Wellingborough: Thorsons, 1982.
3. McIntyre M. *Herbal Medicine for Everyone*. London: Penguin, 1988.
4. Barnard J. *A Guide to the Bach Flower Remedies*. Saffron Walden: CW Daniel, 1987.
5. Chapman JB. *Dr Schluessler's Biochemistry: A Natural Method of Healing*. Wellingborough: Thorsons, 1984.
6. Kenyon J. *21st Century Medicine. A Layman's Guide To The Future*. Wellingborough: Thorsons, 1986.

Section 2

The Homoeopathic Approach to Treating a Patient

9
Seeing the patient: an approach to taking a history

As can be seen from Chapter 4, Hahnemann gave strict instructions on how to take the ideal homoeopathic history (aphorisms 83–103).

In the busy world of primary care it is sometimes difficult to take the long case in one session. Many cases are acute and do not demand a full homoeopathic history. Here a knowledge of the remedies and their modes of action will serve the practitioner well and in this way much first aid advice can be given.

However, for the more chronic case, it is essential that a full history is taken so that the *total symptom picture* is obtained. This is the only way to choose an accurate remedy.

How does one go about advising on a remedy? First, an appropriate history has to be taken. The symptoms are then reviewed and, based on an assessment of the important symptoms, the practitioner will turn to the *repertory*. A repertory is essentially a *materia medica* turned inside out. The latter provides a heading with the name of a remedy, followed by the symptom picture a particular drug is likely to produce. A repertory is a list of symptoms arranged formally, either in book form (Kent or Synthesis) or computerized, with the remedies listed that correspond with the particular symptom.

Homoeopathy does not preclude a full examination and investigating the patient as appropriate. This is where the skills and resources of those working in primary care are such an advantage. Some homoeopaths work in isolation, with little or no medical training and no access to investigations.

Taking a history

The complaint and present symptoms

In general practice we so often hear symptoms that are not significant in conventional medical terms. How often do patients with rheumatic pain mention that the pain is worse only in damp weather, or with the approach of a pressure front? That asthma or chest complaints are worse before a thunderstorm or in wet weather? We tend to ignore these symptoms in normal practice. In homoeopathic medicine these symptoms are invaluable clues in trying to determine the correct remedy.

Although these are most pressing to the patient, it will be seen later that in the assessment of the case and evaluation of symptoms, these symptoms may be less important in the overall selection of the remedy.

Accurate recording of the symptoms is essential. In particular, the speed of development of symptoms will act as a pointer to the type of remedy that may be needed. Precipitants must be ascertained. Was there a previous illness, mental upset or exposure to certain weather conditions before the illness?

The *modalities* must be ascertained. These are factors which affect a symptom and make it worse or better. They are crucial in remedy selection, as two remedies for arthritis, say, may have completely different modalites. For example, Rhus tox. is better for movement, worse for cold, damp weather and better for heat. Bryonia is worse for movement and cold dry weather, especially east winds.

Modalities can usually be classified as:

1. Physical: the effects of posture, position, pressure and movement.
2. Thermal: effects of cold and heat.
3. Weather: effects of weather, be it hot, cold, damp, humid, thunder, sea air or fresh air.
4. Time: many remedies have distinct times when symptoms are worse or better.
5. Laterality: the symptoms may predominate on one side or another or move from side to side.
6. Other: the effect of other factors, i.e. music.

Past medical history

This is as important as, if not more important than, conventional history-taking. If current symptoms can be related to some long forgotten illness, such as prolonged malaise after an attack of glandular fever, then there are clues which may lead us to choose a remedy to treat this past provoking illness – in this case maybe glandular fever nosode. Again, primary care is at an advantage as there is a wealth of information in the patient's notes.

Family history

Important facts can be interpreted in taking a family history. It is crucial that you find out about not just siblings' and parents' health, but even that of the grandparents if possible. The reason for this is that Hahnemann believed that certain traits were inherited and these traits could be treated. A history of tuberculosis, diabetes or cancer is particularly important.

Physical appearance

The physical appearance and manner of the patient may be a clue to that patient's remedy. Although classically described in the texts, in my experience not all 'obsessionally tidy' people are Arsenicum, or slovenly unwashed people Sulphur. Use the appearance as a possible guide, but do not include or exclude symptoms purely on the features you may note.

Generals

These refer to the whole patient and are noted by the patient, who attributes 'I' to the statement about a symptom, e.g. I feel the cold, which is different to a *particular* symptom or presenting complaint, where the patient may prefix the statement by 'my', e.g. my feet are cold.

Ask questions about the following:

1. Temperature: the effect on the patient as a whole. The effect of heat or cold. The symptoms may be further complicated by patients who like a particular condition, but are made worse by it!
2. Weather: the effects of weather are particularly fascinating and in my experience quite prominent in the rheumatic disorders, and in some skin conditions. All types of weather need to be explored; however, it is always more significant if the patient volunteers a particular symptom than if a leading question has been asked.
3. Time: symptoms occurring at particular times may be of significance.
4. Body function: perspiration, urine flow and colour, odour, etc. and bowel action and characteristics of the stool are relevant. Menstrual disturbances may be of great importance and relation of the

symptom to the stage of the cycle – whether premenstrual, during or after menses – is significant.

5. Desires and aversions: again the symptoms are *only significant* if the symptom is strong. Sweet, salt, sour, vinegar, fats, milk and fish are all common. Drinks, particularly quantity and temperature, are significant.
6. Sleep: the pattern of sleep or lack of it! The position in bed and dreams (see section on Mental symptoms) are important.

Do not confuse the above with modalities discussed earlier. A modality is a factor which qualifies a particular symptom, i.e. a 'my' symptom. The above are general symptoms that need to be ascertained about the whole person.

Mental symptoms

As will be seen later, when discussing repertorization and assessing the importance of symptoms, the mentals are the most important group of symptoms. It is the deviation from the normal that is significant.

Questions have to be asked about:

Will	**Understanding**	**Memory**
Anger	Delusions	Forgetfulness
Irritability	Hallucinations	Speech disorders
Sadness	Clairvoyance	Writing disorder
Tendency to cry	Ailments from exertion	
Jealousy		
Indifference		
Suspicion		
Dreams		
Fears		

The first group are the most important, followed by the other two in descending order.

Strange, rare and peculiar

These are symptoms that are unique to a particular case, but in homoeopathy may be the symptoms that would clinch the choice of remedy.

Choosing a remedy

We have taken an exhaustive history, studied the patient and performed an examination. Now comes the possibly more difficult task of choosing the correct remedy. How does one set about doing so?

1. First grade the important symptoms.
2. Use the repertory.
3. Choose the remedy and dose.

Grading the symptoms

Before being able to repertorize you need to assess the symptoms and decide which are the most important.

First, ignore common symptoms. They do not help distinguish one remedy from another. For example, thirst is a common symptom, as is thirst with a fever, but thirst for large quantities of cold drinks, immediately vomited, or thirst with no desire to drink is more significant.

Second, never start with general symptoms such as diarrhoea, headache, etc. They are too general and will have hundreds of remedies in each rubric.

The most important symptoms of the ***first grade*** are the ***mental*** symptoms. If they are marked they will dominate the case. You cannot eliminate these symptoms.

The mentals are graded further:

1. The highest rank is ***will***. This includes love, hate, suspicion and fear, jealousy and relationships with others.
2. The second grade is ***understanding***. This refers to the symptoms related to delusions, perception, delirium, sense of proportion, etc.
3. The third grade is the mentals related to ***memory***.

The next symptoms to identify are those called the ***strange, rare*** and ***peculiar***. These take a high position when choosing significant symptoms. A peculiar mental will outweigh a peculiar local. This is where sometimes they are used in ***keynote*** prescribing.

Keynotes may be invaluable, but only if the generals do not oppose or contradict the remedy choice. Below ***the symptoms are listed*** in order of priority before beginning repertorization.

Next come the ***general*** or ***second-grade*** symptoms. This is how the individual as a whole reacts to the bodily environment. This can be subdivided in order of importance into reactions to bodily environment, cravings and aversions and finally menstrual state.

Finally the particulars are considered. These symptoms are 'my' symptoms, where the patient refers to a particular part.

Summary of grade symptoms

Mentals

Will
Understanding
Memory

Strange, rare, peculiar (if present)

Generals

Reaction of body as a whole to:

Heat and cold
Time
Damp and dry
Atmospheric conditions
Menstruation
Position, motion, pressure
Food aggravation and amelioration
Character of discharges

Physical

Sexual perversions

Stomach

Desires and aversions for foods
Hot and cold foods
Appetite
Thirst

Particulars

Relating to a part, e.g. 'my' symptoms

Paradoxically, the symptoms that are important to the patient and which cause the presentation are not necessarily rated highly when assessing the case and repertorizing. Only those symptoms which are strong are likely to be significant. If a patient volunteers a symptom it is more likely to be of value then one elicited in a trawl of symptoms.

Prescribing

It is important at this stage to realize that there are many ways of selecting a remedy depending on style, time and experience. This is an introductory text emphasizing the importance of *constitutional prescribing*. Constitution is defined as '*the combination of the totality of symptoms combined with the physical characteristics and temperament of the patient*'. There are many cases where time or circumstance does not require a constitutional remedy.

In primary care a number of prescribing styles may be used, especially in acute cases.

These other approaches to the case may include:

1. Keynotes: one or two homoeopathic symptoms are recognized as being characteristic of a certain remedy.
2. Specifics: a single remedy is prescribed for a specific symptom, e.g. arnica for bruising.
3. Epidemic remedy: in an epidemic many cases may respond to one remedy, e.g. gelsemium for flu.
4. Totality of symptoms: the choice is based on the symptoms rather than the constitution; this takes into account physical appearance as well.
5. Miasmatic remedies: a prescription based on the presence of one or a combination of psora, sycosis and syphilis.
6. Never well since: remedies based on an illness at a key point in the patient's past which may have precipitated the present condition.
7. Nosodes: remedies prescribed according to a particular drug picture.
8. Essence: an approach used by Vithoulkas assuming that remedies have themes which may match the patient's symptoms.

There are other styles, including computer choice of remedy, drainage prescriptions and the use of previous successful prescriptions, which may be of value.

Further reading

1. Kent J.T. *Repertory of Homoeopathic Materia Medica*. New Delhi: B Jain Publishers, 1992.

Repertorization

You have graded the symptoms and now have a list of key symptoms. Too many weak symptoms lead to hours of useless searching. Try to choose the strong, high-grade symptoms.

The repertory is a resource which enables one to reference symptoms (rubrics) which will have lists of remedies. The remedies are graded **bold**, *italic* or plain type. This indicates the relative strength and frequency with which that symptom appeared in provings. **Bold** indicates that the symptom occurred in over 80% of provings, *italic* that symptoms appeared in 50% of provings and plain indicates an appearance in provings, but not significantly so.

Kent's repertory, until recently still the most widely used, was first published in 1897. It was Kent's summation of all other repertories to that date, along with his own work and observation. The repertory is divided into 31 sections, beginning with the *mind*, and ending with *generalities*. There is a clear logical pattern to the order of rubrics in any one section.

Kent stresses that studying the repertory is both an art and a science. *One must remember that the purpose of using the repertory is to find the similimum, the most accurate match of remedy with symptomatology.*

There is a logic to the repertory. I still use manual methods as it is a good way of learning about unfamiliar remedies, although there are huge advantages in computerized repertories.

For any symptom the logical progression is always the same:

1. First the *time* at which the symptom occurs.
2. Next the *conditions* under which the symptom has been observed, in alphabetical order.
3. Finally, if the symptom involves *pain*, describe its character, location and onset and its extension.

So, for example, for a patient who is scared of the dark, one would first look at *mind*. Then search *fear*. There will initially be time factors, if relevant to the case. Then search alphabetically for *fear* (dark, p. 43).

For a patient with a stomach pain, cramping in character, which wakes him at 2 a.m., first turn to the section on *stomach*. Then, turning to *pain*, look up the time. Here there are four remedies.

We can further elaborate the symptom as we know the pain is cramping. Turning to *stomach, pain, cramping* (p. 517), we see that there are only two remedies, only one of which appeared in the first group – arsenicum. Knowing the materia medica, one would be able to judge that this is a suitable remedy for this symptom.

Hints on using the repertory

Between the *mentals* at the start and the *generals* at the end are the bulk of symptoms which make up the particulars.

The *generals* section contains the reactions of patients as a whole – the 'I' symptoms. The *generals* section contains much of the pathology of the patient, such as faintness and convulsions. Again, the order for repertorizing remains the same: symptom, then *time*, and associated *conditions* in alphabetical order.

Some *generals* appear in other sections of the book if related to a particular organ: *desires* and *aversions* appear under *stomach*, with *hunger* and *thirst*. These are not the same as aggravations and ameliorations found under the *generals* section. Other *generals* related to menses are found under *genitalia*.

The largest section, extremities, though initially daunting, is still set out in the same logical way: look for the symptom, e.g. *numbness*, followed by the *time*.

Then comes the position in the body, beginning with the *upper limbs, time*, then *condition* and associated factors, covering each section of the upper limb in logical sequence from shoulder to fingers. The pattern is repeated for the *lower limb*.

Pain is dealt with similarly: first the *general* symptom of pain, qualified by *time*. Next there are associated conditions, followed by their location in various parts, e.g. *upper limb, lower limb*.

Then we move to the character of pain. First *generally*; this is searched for alphabetically, from aching to tearing. Then comes the character of the pain in the localities, first upper limb, then lower limb. Then follows the *extension* of the pain. Wherever pain occurs in other sections the pattern is the same.

1. *Pain* generally, with regard to time, and other conditions.

2. *Pain* localized.
3. *Character* of the pain, with time and associated conditions.
4. *Pain* in each locality in turn, with the same breakdown – time, associated conditions and extension.

Only regular use of the repertory and study will enable you to develop a working knowledge of it. Regular usage pays dividends as it helps build up a picture of symptom pictures and unusual rubrics. It also gives you an insight into the smaller remedies which are less often used.

I would strongly recommend reading and rereading Dr Margaret Tyler's excellent article, A study of Kent's repertory[1], to guide you through the process.

Computerized repertories

One only has to look at Kent's repertory or Synthesis to realize that there is a vast amount of data to be reproduced accurately. The size of the book is cumbersome and the material lends itself to computerization. With the availability of affordable hardware and the development of software, homoeopathy is now more than ever accessible on a computer system.

There are many packages available offering a range of facilities, depending on how much the prescriber wants and can afford. The applications are numerous but can be roughly categorized into:

1. Databases of homoeopathic literature.
2. Collection of data from consultations.
3. Computerized repertorizing.

The sheer volume of data a computer is able to store and analyse is phenomenal. Not only can the practitioner access the repertories, but also materia medica can be introduced from different sources to build a picture that fits the patient's needs. It must be noted that the software is not as cheap as other commercial packages, but that reflects the small target market.

Many homoeopaths still rely on manual systems which, although equally useful, are much more time-consuming.

Database of literature

RADAR is the most advanced system of this kind. It was developed between the Faculty of Homoeopathy and the University of Namur in Belgium.

Collection of data from practice

This can be done with most systems. The Faculty of Homoeopathy is collaborating on a project to record symptoms using the READ codes which can then be used for more detailed analysis of the types of cases seen in practice.

Computerized repertorizing

The RADAR package contains Kent's repertory, with synthesis as an option. Rubrics are located by simply typing them.

RADAR offers flexibility when choosing symptoms and their parameters for repertorization. Symptom strength can be graded and this is taken into account when choosing the remedy by computer. RADAR also includes the VES (Vithoulkas expert system), which has been designed to analyse data and produce answers based on the reasoning of an expert in the field, with emphasis given to the mentals.

CARA is a program which uses either Kent or Boericke as a repertory. Remedies are analysed and given scores. It also contains a materia medica.

MAC REPERTORY for Apple Macintosh is in the same format as Kent. Keynotes can be used, and there is a keyword and synonym search. A synthetic repertory includes additions by Eizayaga, Allen, Clarke and Beoricke.

Reference

1. Kent JT. *Repertory of Homoeophathic Materia Medica.* New Delhi: B Jain Publishers, 1992.

11

The first prescription

You have taken a careful history and examined the patient. You are happy with your diagnosis and now want to prescribe. You have therefore selected the key symptoms that make up the case and repertorized and found a remedy, the *similimum*. How do you prescribe, and in what dose?

There are no hard and fast rules. Attend any seminar or discussion group and you will be surprised by the range of approaches that still seem to end in a successful conclusion.

Are there any guidelines on how to prescribe? I think it is fair to say that until it has been proven that there is only one way to prescribe, one can only give general advice on how to approach a case.

If a case has been analysed and you are certain that you have identified a constitutional remedy then you can prescribe a high-potency remedy – 10M. Equally, if the case displays marked mental symptoms, then a high potency is justifiable. If on the other hand the symptoms are local or pathological, then low-potency remedies are suggested, perhaps for several days or even weeks.

There is a grey area in between, where the case may not be totally convincing so the prescriber may be cautious and prescribe a middle-range potency, giving the flexibility to increase or decrease the dose at the next consultation. I use low potency for most general practice patients, and resort to high potency in a 'long case' where I feel there is a clear indication, either in the mentals or the constitution.

To the beginner this may seem vague and imprecise. 'Surely there is a dosage schedule?' a novice may ask. However, as I have stated, there are many approaches to the dose of a medicine and it is only by experience and in some cases trial and error that a prescriber will become confident.

In the primary care setting my advice would be to start with a range of first aid remedies that cover a variety of common complaints until you become familiar with their effects. When you have developed confidence in the use of these remedies it is worth trying other remedies and expanding your therapeutic arsenal gradually in this way. Dr Jack, in his pamphlet, *Introducing Homoeopathy into General Practice*, suggests a starter pack of remedies and this includes Aconite, Belladonna, Ipecac, Arnica, Nux vom., Phosphorus, Ars. alb. and Chamomilla. Dr Jack also dispenses first aid packs to his patients so that they are able to self-administer homoeopathic first aid remedies in the home.

What about side-effects?

Homoeopathic remedies rarely produce side-effects. This is not to say that they do not occur. *Aggravations* occur. There are two principal types of aggravation. In the first there is a worsening of the patient's symptoms followed by a slow improvement in general and mental well-being; this is called a *homoeopathic aggravation.*

Another type of aggravation which may occur is *disease aggravation,* in which a decline in the patient may occur. In the former the remedy chosen was probably correct but in too high a potency; in the latter the remedy was incorrect and the patient needs reassessing.

I give all patients a note warning of the theoretical risk of aggravation, and in such cases to cease therapy immediately until they have spoken to me. In 10 years I can recall only two serious homoeopathic aggravations which settled spontaneously, and three or four disease aggravations. Ernst discusses the issue of safety and side-effects in some detail, and notes that the practitioner is possibly as important a risk in producing problems as the medicine.[1]

Which potency to prescribe?

It is believed that Hahnemann never went above 200C. Theoretically a practitioner could use any potency but over the years guidelines for prescribing have been handed down which are useful to the beginner. Most homoeopaths use the centisimal scale potencies and the M potencies. Experience with LM potencies varies amongst practitioners and I admit to being someone who has never used them.

Low-potency remedies (decimal) and LM potency remedies are repeated more frequently then the centisimal and millesimal M potencies.

As discussed in Chapter 9, there are many approaches to the choice of a remedy – constitutional, epidemic and keynote. Equally, there are various approaches to the taking of the prescription. These include:

1. The single dose: perhaps the ideal, but sometimes not practical. Other approaches may also be needed.
2. The single cumulative dose: increasing potencies of the same remedy until an effect is observed.

3. Split dose: two doses of the same potency given in quick succession. Usually high potencies.
4. Ascending collective dose: increasing potency according to agreed regime of potencies given at intervals and the reaction noted, e.g. 12C, 30C, 200C.
5. Repeated low potencies with accompanying high potency: for example, a constitutional remedy with low potency for specific symptoms.
6. High potency followed by repeated low potencies.

There are other approaches used by homoeopaths with different backgrounds and experience. If the technique works for them then their approach should be respected.

Reference

1. Ernst E. The safety of homoeopathy. *Br Hom J* 1995; **84**: 193–194.

12 The follow-up: case analysis

Kent states that the physician should 'watch and wait and observe'. It is important to keep this rule in mind after the patient has taken a remedy to be able to decide what to do or, more importantly, what not to do. Roberts states that the first prescription is the prescription that first reacts.[1]

What may happen to a patient after taking a prescription? There may be no change, or the remedy given may *aggravate* or *ameliorate* the condition. If the patient has an *aggravation of the disease*, he or she is getting worse. If the patient has an *aggravation of the symptoms*, he or she is getting better. This is when the patient claims that the symptoms are worse, but overall he or she feels better.

It is said that the symptoms that are being removed must be of sufficient depth for a cure to take place. The removal of superficial symptoms *palliates*, but does not cure.

Hering, the prominent American homoeopath, discussed the *directions for cure* which give an indication how a successfully chosen remedy acts:

1. From within, outward.
2. From deep to superficial levels.
3. From above to below.
4. From important organs to the less important.
5. Symptoms disappear in reverse order of their appearance.

These rules help us to assess whether a remedy is having an effect.

In *Lectures on Homoeopathic Philosophy* Kent[1,3] discussed in detail possible outcomes of treatment:

1. Prolonged aggravation and final decline. If this occurs, it indicates that the *vital force* was too weak. Where this may be suspected because the patient is weak, Kent recommends a low-potency remedy.
2. Long aggravation but a slow and final improvement. This may occur when the patient is not as ill as in the above case. Tissue damage may account for the prolonged aggravation.

3. Rapid aggravation with rapid improvement. This is a welcome reaction, implying that the remedy was well-chosen and the patient will do well, as there is no structural damage to the patient's organs.
4. No aggravation. The disease is not of great depth. There is no organic disease and the condition is more likely to be nervous in origin. The potency chosen in this case is exactly right. Kent states that this is the highest order of cure in acute disorders, but also notes that homoeopaths may prefer to see a slight aggravation before cure!
5. Amelioration first, aggravation afterwards. In this case the possibilities are that the remedy was too superficial and only palliated the case, or the patient was incurable and the remedy was suitable.
6. Amelioration, but symptom relief is too short. This may happen in acute cases where the dose has to be repeated several times as the vital force is used up in an acute inflammatory process. In a chronic case it may imply that structural change – damage – is taking place.
7. Permanent amelioration of symptoms, but no special relief. These cases would be considered to be palliated by homoeopathy; because of their particular problems cure cannot be achieved.
8. Proving every remedy. Some patients have an idiosyncracy and are oversensitive. The medicine acts as the disease does.
9. New symptoms appear after the remedy. This implies that the prescription is unfavourable. Make sure that these are new symptoms and not the reappearance of old ones. The latter case implies that a remedy is having an action.
10. Old symptoms reappear. These recurring symptoms are suppressed symptoms that have been replaced by newer ones. This would fit with *Hering's laws of direction of cure* – that symptoms disappear in reverse order of their appearance. No action is taken if the patient is improving.
11. Symptoms take the wrong direction. According to Hering, we hope to see removal of symptoms from the deeper structures to superficial, indicating that a remedy is acting correctly.

Obstacles to cure

Hahnemann discusses this in the *Organon* (aphorisms 252, 253 and 260)[2].

The remedy chosen is the best match for the patient's presenting symptoms. As seen from Kent's descriptions of what may happen when a remedy is taken, there are several possible outcomes.[1,3] When a remedy fails to act, Hahnemann considers that it may not have been the incorrect choice of remedy (although this is possible!), but one or a variety of factors which impeded the homoeopathic remedy's action. These may include poor diet, living conditions, alcohol, smoking, previous illnesses or drugs being taken. Hahnemann also emphasizes the importance of mental health to cure. Stress, negative attitudes, grief and anger can all impair recovery. It is at this point that re-evaluation of not only the problem but also the whole lifestyle may be important.

References

1. Roberts H. *The Principles and art of Cure by Homoeopathy* Chapter XVI. New Delhi: B Jain Publishers, 1988.
2. Hahnemann S. *Organon of Medicine* (Translated by Kunzli, J., Naude, A., Pendleton, P.). London: Victor Gollancz, 1992.
3. Kent JT. *Lectures on Homoeopathic Philosophy*. Worthing: Insight Editions, 1985.

13

The second prescription

The first prescription is the prescription that first reacts. If there is no reaction then it was not the correct prescription.

Kent[1] recommends that a second prescription may be used in the following circumstances:

1. To antidote the first prescription.
2. To complement the first prescription.
3. As a repetition of the first prescription.

Kent urges that in observing the action of a remedy the physician must be patient, watch and wait and observe the action of the first prescription.

Administering a well-chosen remedy too soon after the first dose may make a rational choice of second prescription difficult, as the patient's symptoms may be mixed with drug symptoms. The first prescription should be allowed to work until the patient's symptoms halt. If there is no return of symptoms then there is nothing to do but wait and see if the original symptoms return.

If the first prescription brought long-lasting relief, but then the symptoms returned, this would indicate that the first prescription was correct and can be repeated.

If new symptoms appear after the first prescription and the old symptoms have not returned, then the case must be reviewed. If the symptoms seem similar to those in the drug picture, then the patient may be *proving* the drug. and an *antidote* may be required.

The new remedy must be matched with the new symptoms. If the second prescription must be changed because new symptoms appear, then a new history must be taken and a new second prescription found.

A *complementary* remedy may sometimes be given when a patient takes one remedy successfully for recurring symptoms, but the constitution is not treated. A complementary remedy may be added to complete the case.

There are many examples of relationships between remedies: Belladonna and Calc. carb.; Sulphur, Calc. carb. and Lycopodium; Rhus tox. and Calc. carb., and Bryonia and Natrum mur. are but a few.

Finally, a change of treatment plan may be needed taking into account miasmatic or constitutional features.

References

1. Kent JT. *Lectures of Homoeopathic Philosophy*. Chapters XXXV and XXXVI. Insight Editions. New Delhi: B Jain Publishers, 1988.

Section 3

The Management of Specific Conditions in Primary Care

Disease categories

In Section 3 I have categorized the disease groups commonly seen in general practice and briefly attempted to discuss remedies for each category. No text can be exhaustive and the reader should refer to other texts in addition.

Do not be afraid to experiment. There are many first aid remedies you can cut your teeth on until you have more confidence. I give advice on or prescribe homoeopathy to approximately 10% of all my general practice cases.[1]

I suggest using a limited group of therapies until you become familiar with them. For first aid cases, acute cases and keynote prescribing, the 6C or 30C potency repeated frequently may be appropriate; some experts use 10M for acute treatments.

Availability of remedies can be a factor in choice of potency. Most chemists worth their salt stock remedies in 6C or 30C potency. A container of 125 tablets retails at around £3.50. Experienced practitioners may like to dispense their own medicines using stock bottles containing almost any potency you desire. Practitioners can medicate tablets themselves and give them to the patient.

I have subdivided morbidity according to data provided by the Fourth National Morbidity Study[2] which showed that the most common reasons for consulting were:

Respiratory disease	31%
Nervous system	17%
Musculoskeletal	17%
Skin disorders	15%
Injuries and poisonings	14%
Genito-urinary	11%
Circulatory	9%
Digestive	9%
Mental problems	7%

I have incorporated sections on childhood, pregnancy and district nursing for ease of reference. I have tried to consider the needs of nursing colleagues who may be interested in using homoeopathic remedies. Many of these treatments can be used as self-help remedies. However further experience and training are needed for the most appropriate use of homoeopathy in pregnancy and labour. Section 5 gives an overview of those remedies available, but is not intended to be definitive.

My advice to any practitioner considering using homoeopathy regularly is to attend the excellent introductory courses run by the Faculty at the major centres, Bristol, London and Glasgow, where a thorough grounding is given in the principles of care. The Society of Homoeopaths and British Institute of Homoeopathy mentioned in Appendix 1 also offer innovative teaching programmes.

References

1. Downey P. Audit of prescribing style and outcomes in general practice. *Br Hom J* 1996; **85**: 71–73.
2. Ebrahim S. Changing patterns of consultation in general practice. Fourth morbidity study OPCS. *Br J Gen Pract* 1995; **45**: 395.

15

Respiratory disorders

From the simple management of coughs and colds to more complicated problems such as asthma and allergic problems, homoeopathy can have a part to play. This chapter gives a list of common symptoms and suggested remedies. As with all areas, the doctor will have to consider the patient first and whether homoeopathic treatment is appropriate.

Constitutional prescribing is appropriate for those with recurrent problems.

Common cold

Aconite:	In the early stages, repeated frequently.
Allium cepa:	For sneezing and watery eyes, acrid nasal discharge, bland eye secretion, hot and thirsty, <warm room, > open air.
Arsenicum album:	Watery catarrh, sneezes, burning, very chilly, better for heat.
Gelsemium:	Rapid onset, generalized aches and pains in muscles, running up and down spine, trembling and weakness.
Ferrum phos.:	Pale, chilly (between aconite and gelsemium)
Natrum mur.:	Sneezing in morning, profuse nasal discharge, dry cracked lips (herpes). Irritable. < heat > cool.
Nux vom.:	Irritable, very chilly, shivers if uncovered. Aches all over. > warm drinks and heat. Colds and snuffles. Chilly. Must be covered.
Pulsatilla.:	Catarrh, thick, bland and yellow. Thirstless, chilly. < heat > fresh air.

Influenza

Aconite:	Especially after exposure to cold; use in first stages.
Baptisia:	Septic conditions, muscular soreness, with offensive secretions. Mentally confused, stupor.
Bryonia:	Aching in every muscle, stitching pains which are worse for movement. Dry membranes. Irritable. Splitting headache.
Camphor:	First stages of cold with chilliness and sneezing. Exposure to chill. Icy coldness of body.
Eupatorium:	For flu with bone pain. Aching in bones with soreness of flesh and muscles. < night.
Gelsemium:	Drowsiness, dullness and trembling. Muscular weakness. Eyelids heavy. Flushed face. Hot dry skin. Better for urination.
Pyrogen:	Restlessness, septic states. Offensive discharges. Bursting headache. Dry red tongue. Palpitations.

It may be worth considering the Influenzinum nosode as a preventative, or for people with slow recovery after influenza.

Coughs and upper respiratory tract infections

Aconite:	Always of use in the early stages of a cold or flu. If not aborted by aconite then another remedy will need to be considered. Sudden onset. Restless and anxious. Thirst for cold drinks. < warm room. Bounding pulse.
Antimonium tart.:	Rattling chest, cold, sweaty, little expectoration. Tongue dry but thirstless. Stuporose. Sometimes used in left ventricular failure for chest symptoms.
Bryonia:	Dry cough, stitching pains in chest. < movement > rest>. pressure on affected side. Dry lips. Thirst cold drinks. Right-sided chest symptoms.
Causticum:	After exposure to cold, frosty weather. Hoarseness, dryness, rawness in trachea and loss of voice. > sips of cold water. Pale thin sallow appearance.
Drosera:	Paroxysmal cough. Of value in pertussis. Chilly.

	Perspires ++. Sneezing. Hoarseness. Violent cough < lying down at 2 a.m.
Ipecac:	Chilly, sudden onset of respiratory symptoms. Rattling of chest, associated with nausea unrelieved by vomiting. Constriction of chest and incessant cough.
Kali. carb.:	Chilly, stitching pains. 3 a.m. aggravation. Weary. Weakness, paroxysmal cough, wheeze, > sitting forward. Yellow catarrh.
Phosphorus:	Hoarseness. Pain in larynx. Tickling cough. Worse for cold air. Tightness and weight across chest. Worse lying on left side.
Rumex: (yellow dock)	Cough, tickling, worse for slightest draught of cold air.
Spongia:	Dryness, hoarseness. Dry barking croupy cough. Panting respiration. < lying down with head low.

Throat problems

Acute attacks recurring on a frequent basis may need investigation. A constitutional remedy or a nosode may also be of value.

Calc. carb.:	Fat, fair and chilly. Large glands. Stitches on swallowing.
Hepar sulph.:	Inflammation. Yellow exudate. Sensation of plug when swallowing. Stitching pain extends to ear when swallowing.
Lachesis:	Sore, worse left side, when swallowing liquids. Dry throat aggravated by hot drinks. Painful, worse for pressure. Purplish tonsils. Worse swallowing saliva. Pain extends to ear. Dislikes tight collar around neck.
Lycopodium:	Dry, thirstless. Stitches on swallowing, but better for warm drinks. Suppuration beginning on right side. Worse cold drinks.
Merc. sol.:	Bluish red swelling. Desire to swallow. Putrid throat. Worse on right. Stitching pain referred to ear. Raw burning offensive. Loss of voice.
Nitric acid:	Dry sensation of splinters in throat when swallowing.

Phytolacca:	Dark red or bluish. Sensation of lump in throat. Swollen tonsils, especially right side. Pain shoots to ears. Greyish membrane across throat. Cannot swallow anything hot. Mumps.

Croup

Aconite:	Early stage of any upper respiratory tract infection, especially after exposure to cold air.
Antimonium tart.:	Rattling chest. Sits up.
Hepar sulph.:	Hoarse, cough, worse when exposed to cold. Loose rattling cough worse in morning and after midnight.
Kali. carb.:	Worse lying on right and at 3 a.m. Leaning forward relieves symptoms. Wheeze.
Spongia:	Hoarse, dryness of tubes. Barking cough. Croup worse for inspiration and before midnight. Better after eating or drinking.

Hay fever

There are a variety of remedies which are useful for a range of specific symptom pictures. There are also a number of allergens in potentized form which can be used in the treatment of the specific allergy.

Allium cepa:	Bland lacrimation and acrid nasal discharge. Worse warm room. Better in open air.
Arsenicum alb.:	Burning eyes, acrid lacrimation. Oedema around eyes. Thin watery excoriating discharge. Sneezing without relief.
Arsenicum iod.:	More corrosive discharges. Constant desire to sneeze.
Arundo:	Burning and itching of palate and conjunctiva. Itching of nostrils and the roof of the mouth.
Euphrasia:	Profuse lacrimation, better in open air. Acrid lacrimation, bland coryza. Eyes water all the time.
Pulsatilla:	Thick profuse, bland yellow discharge. Itching and burning of eyes. Lids inflamed and agglutinated. Loss of smell.

Sabadilla:	Eyelids red and burning. Profuse lacrimation. Spasmodic sneezing.
Allergens:	Allergens to consider for hay fever like symptoms, taken up to a month or so before the expected season are useful.
	Birch pollen in April, grass pollen in May/June, mould and grass pollens in the autumn is a common sequence depending on the patient's susceptibility. The manufacturers will supply you with lists of available allergens in potentized form. Other allergens that cause similar symptoms all year round may be tried if a source of the irritation can be identified. Consider cat dander, dust mite or horse fur for the respective allergic conditions.

Asthma

Antimonium tart.:	Rattling of mucus. Wheeze. Little expectoration.
Arsenicum alb.:	Wheezing, worse at midnight. Restless. Suffocative catarrh.
Ipecac:	Dyspnoea and constriction in chest. Incessant cough. Persistent cough.
Kali carb.:	Cutting pains in chest. Cough at 3 a.m. with stitching pains. Eased by leaning forward.
Phosphorus:	Cough, worse from cold air. Tightness and weight across chest. Worse on lying on left side.

Miscellaneous problems

Earache

Belladonna:	Throbbing, heat and redness.
Chamomilla:	Angry child. One cheek red and hot. Drives patient frantic.
Graphites:	Chilly. Offensive discharge. Cracking of skin. Fissures.
Hepar sulph.:	Pustules in canal. Fetid pus.
Merc. sol.:	Pain worse in warm bed. Fetid discharge.

Pulsatilla:	Thick, bland offensive odour.
Sulphur:	Meatus, red and itchy.

Catarrh

A full history will be needed in cases of long duration. The use of constitutional remedies and nosodes may be considered.

Kali bich.:	Snuffles in children. Pressure and pain at root of nose. Thick ropy green yellow discharge. Tough plugs of mucus.
Natrum mur.:	Violent coryza. Thin watery discharge. Early stages of cold with sneezing.

Accidents and emergencies/Eye problems

General practice sees its fair share of injuries and trauma. This chapter deals with the common injures and their treatment. It is not meant to be exhaustive, and will not replace experience. Many of these are first aid remedies. Unless otherwise stated, a dose of 6C or 30C repeated frequently is adequate. Some authorities advocate the use of ascending potencies, e.g. 6C, 30C, 200C, 10M, whilst others recommend 10M alone.

Bruising:	Arnica.
Crush injury:	Hypericum where there is damage to the nerve endings.
Fractures:	Arnica, or aconite for physical and mental shock respectively. Symphytum for improved bone healing.
Sprains:	Arnica for bruising. Rhus tox. for pain.
Synovitis:	Rhus tox.
Periosteal pain/ ligament injuries:	Ruta.
Muscular injury/ strain:	Arnica, Rhus tox.
Head injury:	Arnica. Consider Natrum sulph. for delayed effects of injury.
Heat stroke:	Glonoinum or belladonna.
Exhaustion:	Arnica.
Stings/bites:	Ledum is good for puncture wounds. Apis mel for stings. Urtica urens for urticarial wheals.
Wounds:	Use Arnica for trauma, Calendula lotion for wounds. Staphysagria for postop wound pain.
Blisters:	Causticum internally. Cantharis for burns or scalds.

Conjunctivitis

Aconite:	Feel dry and hot. Lids swollen, hard and red. Photophobia, worse after exposure to dry cold winds. After extraction of foreign bodies from eye.
Arg. nit.:	Inner canthi swollen and red. Profuse pus. Chronic ulceration of lids. Eye strain from close work. Worse in warm room.
Arsenicum alb.:	Burning with acrid lacrimation. Intense photophobia, restless and irritable.
Euphrasia:	Cattarhal conjunctivitis with acrid lacrimation. Water all the time. Thick and excoriating.
Pulsatilla:	Thick yellow discharge. Bland. Itching and burning. Styes.
Silica:	Swelling of lacrimal duct. Aversion to light. Styes and iritis. Abscess on cornea after traumatic injury.

Black eye

Arnica:	For initial bruising and after injury.
Ledum:	Extravasation of blood into lids, conjunctiva, aqueous and vitreous.
Symphytum:	Where there is bony damage to the orbit.

Iritis

Hepar sul.:	Ulcers on cornea, profuse discharge and sensitivity to cold and air. Lids red and inflamed. Pain in orbits.
Merc. sol.:	Profuse burning, acrid discharge. Floating black spots. After exposure to glare of fire, arc eye.
Merc. corr.:	Pain behind eyeballs, acrid lacrimation and photophobia. Lids oedematous and red.

Meibomian cysts

Consider the use of thuja or staphysagria.

Styes

Pulsatilla, graphites and sulphur are useful.

17

Musculoskeletal symptoms: a guide for the GP and physiotherapist

Musculoskeletal problems constitute a large part of the work of primary health care, injuries and back pain account for a large proportion of these.

Rather than concentrate on disease syndromes, such as rheumatoid arthritis, it is easier to concentrate on the symptoms, such as joint pain and muscle stiffness. Even within even these two symptom groups there is much scope for discussion of the wide range of remedies which can be tried.

The place of diet, anti-inflammatories and other complementary therapies depends on the views of the practitioner and patient. Where appropriate, and with the patient's agreement, I use acupuncture, diet and physiotherapy and am happy for patients to experiment with regimes which suit them and will do no harm.

Joint pain

Apis mel:	Swollen and red. Better for cool and worse for touch and pressure.
Arnica:	When injury may have preceded pain in affected joint.
Bryonia:	For acute pain. No relief from movement, better for rest and pressure and cold applications.
Calc. phos.:	Rheumatic pains from draught of air. Soreness in sacroiliac joint. Stiffness and pain with cold numb feeling. Worse with any change in weather.
Causticum:	Tearing pains in joints. Contracted tendons. Better for warmth. Better in damp wet weather. Worse in dry cold winds.
Colchicum:	Joints stiff and feverish. Shifting rheumatism. Gout. Cannot bear to be touched. Worse from sundown to sunrise. Worse for motion.
Dulcamara:	Rheumatism alternates with diarrhoea and after

acute skin eruptions. Worse in cold damp rainy weather.

Eupatorium perf.: Bone pain. Aching in bones, arms and wrist with soreness of flesh.

Ledum: Gouty pains, especially in small joints of foot. Begins in lower limbs and ascends. (Opposite of Kalmia.)

Pulsatilla: Restlessness. Pains shift rapidly. Better for slow movement and cool applications.

Rhus tox.: Hot painful joints. Tearing in tendons, ligaments and fascia. Stiff limbs. Worse for cold damp weather and rain and during rest.

Ruta: Acts on periosteum and cartilage. For effects of strain of flexor tendons. Bruised bones. Restlessness. Worse for cold wet weather.

Back pain

Arnica: Sprained and dislocated feeling. Soreness after overexertion. Bed feels too hard.

Arsenicum album: Weakness and burning in small of back. Restless.

Calc. carb.: Pain as if sprained, pain from overlifting. Pain between shoulder blades. Curve of thoracic vertebrae. Stiff neck.

Nux vom.: Lumbar backache. Burning pain, worse between 3 and 4 a.m. Must sit up to turn in bed.

Rhus tox.: Pain and stiffness in small of back, better in motion, worse for lying on something hard.

Muscular pains

Arnica: Pains in back as if bruised and beaten. Sprained feeling. Soreness after overexertion. Bed too hard. Rheumatism begins low down and spreads upwards. Worse for touch, motion and damp cold.

Bryonia: Worse on least movement. Every spot is painful on pressure.

Ledum: Rheumatism that begins in lower limbs and ascends.

Rhus tox.:	Tearing pains in joints, ligaments and tendons. Better for movement. Rhuematic pains spread over nape of neck and down back. Limbs stiff. Worse for cold. Trembling after exertion.
Ruta:	Spine and limbs feel bruised. Tendons sore. Thigh pains when stretching the limbs.

Other remedies to consider include Causticum, Colchicum and Pulsatilla.

Bone pain

Aurum met.:	Pains in bones of head. Exostoses. Worse at night. Dull tearing pains. Debilitating.
Eupatorium perf.: (Thoroughwart)	Bone pains after flu. Pains in bones from secondaries. Aching with soreness of muscles.
Kali. bich.:	Pains move rapidly from one place to another. Worse for cold. Better for motion. Tearing pains in the tibia. Pains in small spots.
Phosphorus:	Burning pains in bones.
Rhododendron:	Acute joint and bone pains. Rheumatic tearing in all limbs. Worse at rest and stormy weather. Pains in spots.
Ruta:	Restlessness, associated pains in tendons.
Silica:	Sciatica. Thin weak children.
Syphilinum:	Severe pain in long bones. Muscles caked in hard lumps.

Sciatica

Colocynth:	Left-sided. Drawing, tearing pain, better for pressure and heat. Worse for gentle touch.
Kali. carb.:	Small of back feels weak. Burning in spine with sudden sharp pains extending down back and to thighs.
Mag. phos.:	Sciatica, feet very tender. Right-sided. Neuralgic pain relieved by warmth.
Rhus tox.:	Pain and stiffness in small of back. Better for motion or lying on something hard.

The nervous system and mental health

Whilst many neurological and psychological cases can be helped by homoeopathy, the chronic nature of the condition makes them difficult to treat. A long case approach is necessary and a constitutional remedy with remedies for local symptoms may be required. Similarly, psychological cases may need a constitutional case, although some conditions can benefit from the use of keynote remedies.

Mental symptoms appear in the Mind section of the repertory. To illustrate the need choose the right remedy, there are 37 **bold**-type remedies under the heading Anxiety and a further 87 in *italic* type.

Like all the conditions listed, these lists are not and cannot be exhaustive. Study of the repertory will increase the number of remedies of possible use to you.

Anger

Aconite:	Resulting from fright or shock.
Chamomilla:	In young children, teething and colic. One flushed cheek.
Colocynth:	Anger accompanied by neuralgia or colic.
Ignatia:	Anger leading to hysterical reactions.
Nux vomica:	Irritability and anger. Overstressed, overworked men.
Staphysagria:	Suppressed anger, leading to physical and emotional symptoms.

Concussion

Arnica:	Following trauma.
Hypericum:	If the head is sensitive.
Natrum sulph.:	For delayed recovery after head injury and mental confusion resulting from trauma.

Delirium

Aconite:	With fear.
Arsenicum:	Worse after midnight, prostration and restlessness.
Belladonna:	Flushed red skin. Fever.
Hyoscyamus:	Suspicious, laughs at everything. Attempts to run away. Mania. Talkative.
Lachesis:	Talkative, suspicious, jealous. Worse in the morning. Loses sense of time.
Stramomium:	Ceaseless talking. Swearing, praying, delusions and hallucinations. Violent. Religious mania. Needs light and company. Desire to escape.

Depression (rubric = sadness)

Anacardium:	Depressed and irritable. Lacks self-confidence. Desire to swear and curse. Feels possessed. Two wills.
Arsenicum album:	Restless, nightly aggravation. Anguish. Fears death. Feels it is useless to take medicine. Sadness drives the person from place to place.
Aurum metallicum:	Hopeless, despondent and wants to commit suicide. Disgust for life. Talks of suicide. Oversensitive to noise.
Calc. Carb.:	Depression due to overwork. Apprehensive. Fears. Forgetful and confused.
Ignatia:	Changeable mood, introspective. Contradictory. Sighing and sobbing. After grief and for hysteria.
Lycopodium:	Melancholy, dislikes being alone. Apprehensive.
Natrum mur.:	Effects of grief or fright. Consolation aggravates. Wants to be alone to cry. Tears with laughter.
Phosphoric acid:	Indifferent. Listless.
Pulsatilla:	Changeable. Weeps easily. Fear in the evening.
Sulphur:	Selfish. Irritable and depressed.

Fear

Aconite:	Effects of fright, shock. Acute remedy only.

Argent nit.:	Anticipatory fear with diarrhoea.
Phosphorus:	Fear of being alone, dark and thunder.
Pulsatilla:	Full of fears with weeping.

Headaches including migraine

Arnica:	After head injury.
Belladonna:	Throbbing, bursting headache with flushed appearance and dilated pupils.
Bryonia:	Better for pressure and rest. Bursting, splitting headache. Worse motion. (Acute of Natrum mur.)
Gelsemium:	Dull heavy ache with heaviness of eyelids. Band-like feeling and occipital headache. Pain in temple extending to ear. Preceded by blindness and relieved by urination.
Glonoine:	Throbbing headache after exposure to the sun.
Lycopodium:	Worse from 4 to 8 p.m. Better uncovered. Occipital tearing pain. Right-sided.
Mag. phos.:	Neuralgic pain. Right side. Better for warmth.
Nat. mur.:	Blinding headache. Semilateral. Hammering inside skull. Worse after menses, and between sunrise and sunset. Nausea and vomiting.
Nux vomica:	Perioral tingling precedes. Relieved by sleep. Occipital headache with vertigo. Worse for stimulants. Post-hangover remedy.
Sanguinaria:	Right-sided. Periodical sick headache. From occiput it spreads over scalp and settles over eyes, especially right. Pain better lying down and after sleep.

Hypochondriasis

Arsenicum album:	With depression. Prostration out of proportion to problem.
Aurum net.:	Black despair. Suicidal ideas.
Calc. carb.:	Anxiety with palpitations. Fears loss of reason.
Ignatia:	Hysterical

Impaired memory

Aethusa cynapium:	Inability to think or fix attention. Associated intolerance of milk. Brain fag.
Bartya carb.: (barium)	Mental weakness and loss of memory. Disorders of old age. Swollen glands.
Conium:	Weak memory of elderly. Weakness of body with trembling.
Lycopodium:	Weak memory. Confused thoughts. Spells or writes wrong words.
Sulphur:	Forgetful. Lazy. Delusion of greatness. Peevishness.

Neuralgia

Aconite:	Neuralgia, especially left side with associated numbness and tingling. After exposure to cold.
Actaea racemosa:	Like electric shocks. Associated anxiety. Widespread pains that come and go.
Arsenicum alb.:	Intermittent burning pains. Irritability and anxiety.
Colocynth:	Irritable, easily angered. Cutting twisting pains relieved by pressure. Left-sided facial pain.
Kalmia:	Right-sided facial pain. Stitches. Shift rapidly. Pain shoots downwards with numbness.
Mag. phos.:	Spasm, relieved by warmth, rubbing and pressure. Colic relieved by bending forward. Right-sided.
Spigelia:	Semi-lateral pain. Left side.

Panic

Aconite:	After shock
Argentum nit.:	Fearful and nervous. Anticipatory anxiety.
Arsenicum:	Fear of being alone.
Gelsemium:	Stage fright.
Lycopodium:	Apprehensive. Fear of being alone, yet dislikes company.

Sleep problems (24 pages in repertory, including dreams)

Aconite:	Restless disturbed sleep.
Arnica:	Bed feels hard.
Coffea:	Wakeful and restless. Sleeps until 3 a.m. then only dozing. Sleeplessness because of mental activity. Flow of ideas.
Kali. carb.:	Wakes at 3 a.m. and cannot return to sleep.
Lycopodium:	Drowsy during day.
Phosphorus:	Sleeplessness in elderly. Vivid dreams and nightmares.
Sulphur:	Cat-nap type sleep. Worse for heat.

Vertigo

Borax:	Dread of downward motion.
Calc. carb.:	Vertigo on ascending and when turning head.
Cocculus:	Vertigo with nausea when riding or sitting up.
Nux vom.:	Vertigo with momentary loss of consciousness. Intoxicated feeling. Worse in morning.

Stroke

Arnica:	After-effect of injury or bruise to brain.
Natrum sulph.:	Ill effect of falls or injuries to head.
Opium:	Drowsiness. Dull heavy stupid sleep.

19

Skin problems

Skin problems represent a significant part of the work of general practice. Resistant cases requiring the frequent use of antibiotics or steroids tend to be the ones referred to the homoeopath as a last resort! There are many minor conditions that may be helped by these remedies.

It is important to look for a constitutional remedy wherever possible. Miasmatic prescribing strategies are likely to be of use in skin disorders.

Acne

Belladonna:	Dry, hot and swollen. Pustules on face. Boils.
Calc. silicata.:	Itching, burning, cold and blue. Comedones. Chilly.
Calc. sulph.:	Unhealthy discharging skin. Yellow crusts and scabs.
Hepar sulph.:	Chilly. Suppuration. Acne. Pustules.
Pulsatilla:	Acne at puberty, in fair skinned types.
Silica:	Abscesses and slow healing of lesions.
Staphylococcin:	Prominence of pustules and slow response to indicated remedy.
Sulphur:	Dry, scaly and unhealthy. Itching worse for washing.

Blisters

Cantharis:	Vesicular eruptions with itching and burning, relieved by cold applications.
Lachesis:	Hot skin. Blisters have bluish purple appearance. Dark blisters.
Mezereum:	Intolerable itch. Ulcers itch and burn and are

	surrounded by blisters. Scabs with purulent matter beneath.
Nat. mur.:	Greasy skin. Crusty eruptions in bends of skin, margins of scalp and behind ears.
Ranunculus:	Burning and intense itching. Herpetic eruptions, especially thoracic zoster. Bluish vesicles in zoster. Blister-like eruptions in palms.
Rhus tox.:	Red, swollen with intense itch. Chickenpox.

Boils

Apis:	Sore and sensitive. Carbuncles with burning, stinging pain.
Belladonna:	Hot, red and throbbing. Worse for touch.
Graphites:	Fat chilly individuals. Unhealthy skin; every injury suppurates.
Hepar sulph.:	Chilly individuals. Prone to abscesses and boils which suppurate. Cannot bear being uncovered.
Lachesis:	Hot skin. Boils have purplish appearance.
Merc. sol.:	Moist skin, with offensive odour. Vesicular and pustular eruptions. Glands swell every time patient takes a cold.
Silica:	Delicate and pale individual with pale waxy skin. Every injury suppurates.
Sulphur:	Dry scaly skin. Worse for washing. Hot. Itching and burning lesions.
Tarentula: (cubensis)	Red spots and pimples. Carbuncles with a purplish hue. Abscesses where pain and inflammation predominate.

Burns and scalds

Sterile dressing soaked in hypercal or urtica urens topically may help. Mix tincture in water. Suggested 20–30 drops in half a litre of water. Calendula lotion may be applied topically.

Cantharis:	Burning and scalding with rawness, relieved by cold applications.

Causticum:	Old burns that do not heal well. Pain from burns. Cicatrices may soften with treatment.
Urtica:	Urticaria, itching blotches. Swelling of tissues with redness.

Chilblains

Agaricus:	Burning itching of extremities. Like frostbite. Swollen veins with cold skin.
Apis:	Redness with swelling of extremities. Worse for heat. Burning stinging pain.
Petroleum:	Dry sore and leathery skin. Cracks worse in winter.
Pulsatilla:	Chilliness, worse in warm rooms.

Eczema

Alumina:	Intolerable itching when warm in bed. Dry and scaly skin.
Arsenicum alb.:	Itching burning and swelling of skin. Dry rough and scaly, worse for cold. Useful in psoriasis.
Graphites:	Rough, dry, hard skin. Eruptions ooze a sticky yellow fluid. Rawness if flexures. Every injury suppurates. Worse for warmth.
Hepar sulph.:	Unhealthy skin which suppurates easily. Sensitive to cold. Very chilly.
Kali. sulph.:	Profuse desquamation. Psoriasis and eczema. Burning itching eruptions, worse in warm room, better in cool air.
Mezereum:	Eczema with intolerable itching. Worse in bed. Exudate sometimes in crust under plaques of skin.
Petroleum:	Dry, constricted and roughened skin. Crusts which crack and bleed. Worse for damp and in winter.
Radium brom.:	Erythema and redness with burning and itching. As if skin on fire. (I have used this in cases of post-radiotherapy erythema and eczema.)
Rhus tox.:	Red, swollen and itching with tendency to vesicle formation.

Sulphur:	Dry and unhealthy skin. Hot red and burning. Worse at night and in bed. Worse for washing.

Lymphadenopathy

Obviously local causes or more sinister pathology must be considered in all instances. There are however patients with persistently enlarged glands, or whose glands enlarge with each minor cold or illness.

Barium carb.:	Especially in infancy and old age. Always has swollen tonsils. Takes cold easily, suppurating tonsils from every cold.
Calc. carb.:	Antipsoric remedy. Takes cold easily and sensitive to cold. Swelling of tonsils and neck glands. Inguinal glands can be painful.
Conium:	Glandular tissue enlarges and becomes painful. Breasts tender before menses. Glands indurated. Night sweats.
Silica:	Every injury suppurates. Indurated tumours. Lesions slow to heal.

Urticaria

Most cases will be ameliorated by either Apis mel or Urtica urens as a first aid remedy. Further questioning and repertorization may be needed for more complex cases.

Genito-urinary conditions

Whilst many of these problems in this chapter are primarily related to female conditions, I have chosen a few specific to men also.

It is estimated that genito-urinary problems account for 9% of consultations in general practice. To many of my female colleagues this may seem a gross underestimate, judging by the comments I hear about the volume of gynaecological problems they see.

The conditions listed below are common, and seem to respond well to homoeopathic treatment.

Cystitis

Obviously when tackling this problem one has to exclude infection and other renal pathology. Patients with recurrent symptoms sometimes carry an indicated remedy with them.

Cantharis:	Intolerable urging and tenesmus. Bloody urine. Paroxysms of cutting and burning in whole renal region. Urine leaks in drops and scalds. Constant desire to urinate.
Causticum:	Involuntary leakage when coughing or sneezing. Expelled slowly; sometimes retention after operation. Loss of sensibility on passing urine.
Clematis:	Tingling in urethra some time after urinating. Interrupted flow. Urethra feels constricted. Inability to pass all the urine; it flows drop by drop.
Equisetum:	Effect mainly on bladder. Dull pain and feeling of fullness in bladder. Frequent urging with severe pain at the close of urination. Urine flows drop by drop. Sharp burning and cutting pains.
Pulsatilla:	Increased desire when lying down. Burning in urethra and during micturition.

Sarsparilla:	Scanty, slimy and bloody urine. Renal colic. Pain at end of micturition. Urine dribbles while sitting. Poor thin stream.
Staphysagria:	Urgency in newly married; 'honeymoon cystitis'. Sensation as if a drop of urine is continually rolling along. Burning in urethra when not urinating. Urging and pain after urinating.
Terebinth:	Strangury with bloody urine. Odour of violets! Urethritis with painful erections and constant tenesmus.

Menstrual disorders

Painful periods (dysmenorrhoea)

Belladonna:	Sensitive genitalia, as if all viscera would prolapse. Cutting pain with bright red loss. Breasts feel heavy, hard and red.
Caulophyllum: (blue cohosh)	Rigid os causing severe cramping pains. Menses and leukorrhoea profuse.
Chamomilla:	Impatient, irritable and hot. Profuse dark clotted blood. Labour-like pains which spread upwards.
Cimcifuga:	Pain before menses. Profuse dark coagulated blood with backache. Afterpains with sensitivity.
Mag. phos.:	Menstrual colic. Dark and stringy loss.
Pulsatilla:	Late menses, thick dark, clotted. Chilly with sensation of downward pressure. Back pain.
Sepia:	Bearing-down sensation: patient crosses the legs to prevent the feeling. Menses early and profuse, or late and scanty. Violent stitching pain from vagina up to umbilicus.

Heavy periods (menorrhagia)

Belladonna:	Bright red, too early and profuse. Offensive discharge.
Calc. carb.:	Profuse heavy menses. Chilly. Premenstrual symptoms. Cutting pains in uterus. Increased sexual desire. Breasts tender and swollen before menses.

China:	Menses early, profuse with heavy clots and abdominal distension. Profuse pain. Heaviness in pelvis.
Ferrum met.:	Menses profuse. Too early and too long. Watery. Sensitive vagina.
Ipecac:	Profuse and gushing with nausea. Pain from navel to uterus.
Sabina:	Special action on uterus. Profuse bright menses. Pain from sacrum to pubis. Haemorrhage partly clotted; worse on movement.
Secale:	Menstrual colic. Intolerant of heat. Irregular profuse menses with oozing of watery blood.
Sepia:	Bearing-down pains. Can have early and profuse menses in sepia types.

Premenstrual syndrome

I have found homoeopathy useful in premenstrual syndrome. I also give advice on other complementary approaches, including the use of vitamin B_6, diet and lifestyle adjustments.

Just as in other 'female' complaints, similar remedies are used repeatedly, as the symptom picture is so broad.

A constitutional remedy may be required, although the symptoms can sometimes be removed using only specifics which fit the picture.

Calc. carb.:	Fat, flabby and chilly. Apprehensive. Headache, colic and leukorrhoea before menses.
Lachesis:	Loquacious. Jealous. Palpitations and breast pain. Hot. All symptoms relieved by the flow.
Lilium:	'Hot Sepia'. Bearing-down sensation with profuse menses. Sensation of prolapse. Bloated feeling. Depression of spirits. Desire to weep constantly.
Natrum mur.:	Coldness. Dry mucous membranes. Weakness and weariness. Consolation aggravates. Headache, after menstruation. Hot during menses.
Pulsatilla:	Tired and weepy. Changeable. Likes sympathy.
Sepia:	Bearing-down sensation. Painful menses. Weak and chilly. Indifferent to loved ones.

Vaginal discharge

Kreosotum:	Corrosive itching. Burning and swelling of vulva. Yellow acrid discharge. Worse between periods.
Mercurius:	Excoriating offensive discharge with sensation of rawness of parts.
Medorrhinum:	Intense pruritus. Thin excoriating discharge with fishy odour.
Nitric acid:	Sore labia with ulcers. Brown watery discharge.
Pulsatilla:	Thick bland green-yellow discharge.
Sepia:	Bearing-down sensation. Yellow-green discharge with much itching.

The menopause

The menopause can present as a wide array of symptoms, including vaginal and skin dryness, flushes, joint pains, headaches and lethargy and feeling generally unwell.

Listed below are a few of the commonly used remedies which fit a variety of symptom pictures. However a constitutional remedy may be required.

Belladonna:	Hot. Irregular heavy menses. Genitalia feel heavy. Flushes of face. Red and congested.
Lachesis:	Hot, loquacious. Irritable. Mood swings. Flushes. All symptoms relieved by menstrual flow.
Lilium tigrinum:	(Hot sepia.) Depression. Worried. Palpitations. Tight chest. Bearing-down sensation. Bloated feeling.
Sepia:	Bearing-down sensation. Indifferent to loved ones. Weepy. Hot flushes and easy perspiration.
Pulsatilla:	Peevish, chilly, weepy. Mood changes. Fears. Melancholy.

Male urinary problems

Prostatism

A thorough investigation of the urinary tract is needed for men presenting with persistent urinary symptoms. I have found homoeopathy useful in treating some of the troublesome symptoms of prostatism. This does not preclude the patient being investigated.

Bartya carb.:	Urge to urinate. Enlarged prostate. Burning in urethra.
Conium:	Increased desire. Power decreased. Difficulty in voiding; starts and stops again.
Iodum:	Indurated gland. Frequent urine.
Pulsatilla:	Increased desire. Burning in urethral orifice. Involuntary micturition while coughing. Discharge from urethra. Prostatitis.
Sabal serrulata:	Enuresis. Enlargement of prostate.

21

The cardiovascular system

The Office of Population Censuses and Surveys[1] survey of GPs' workload suggests that only 9% of activity is related to cardiovascular problems. This is surprising considering the number of people with hypertension who are seen and checked regularly.

I have to confess that this group of medicines is the one I have used least. Many of the patients I see are already taking or have been commenced on powerful drugs which act on the cardiovascular system, and I have found it difficult to introduce homoeopathic remedies in everyday general practice. Where I have used homoeopathic remedies at the patient's request it has been with varying success.

There are several helpful articles on this subject.[2]

Angina

Aconite:	Anxiety and tension after onset of pain with palpitations.
Cactus:	Angina with cold sweat and tight band around chest. Pain shooting into left arm.
Kalmia:	Dyspnoea and pressure from epigastrium up to heart. Sharp pains take the breath away. Pains down left side. Associated slow pulse.
Lilium tigrinum:	Grasping pain which comes and goes. Bearing-down sensation in pelvic viscera. Very hysterical person. Hot and hurried.
Spigelia:	Palpitations. Stabbing pain, which radiates down either arm. Worse for motion and sitting down. Fear of pins. Neuralgic pain.

Arrhythmias

Holland[2] suggests that constitutional treatment is most useful. Other useful remedies include aconite after shock and arsenicum album when there is restlessness and palpitations with pain and associated prostration. Natrum mur. may be a useful remedy for arrhythmias.

Heart failure

Blackie suggests that for acute heart failure the three remedies to consider are Arsenicum album, Antimonium tart. and Carbo. veg.[3]

Antimonium tart.: Palpitations with uncomfortable hot feeling. Rattling mucus in chest, but not as anxious as arsenicum. Thirstless with oedema of lungs.

Carbo. veg.: Mentally and physically exhausted. Bluish appearance, generally collapsed state. Distended and flatulence. Icy cold.

For heart failure of slow onset other remedies include:

Lachesis: Cannot stand any pressure around throat. Hot. Sensation of suffocation. Rushes for open window. Needs to take a deep breath. Associated jealousy and loquacity.

Laurocerasus: Chronic cyanotic disease. Cough and dyspnoea worse sitting up. Worse for exertion. Jelly-like expectoration.

Lycopus: Lowers blood pressure. Praecordial chest pain, constriction and tenderness. Associated with thyroid disease.

Convallaria (lily of the valley) and cratageus are both used in heart failure in the mother tincture formulation.

Hypertension

Rather than listing specific suitable remedies, the constitutional remedies will probably be of most use here. Clarke[4] mentions Aconite, Veratrum viride and Viscum album in tincture. I have used Natrum mur. and Sulphur with minor or no significant success.

References

1. Ebrahim S. Changing patterns of consultation in general practice: fourth national morbidity study 1991–1992. *Br J Gen Prac* 1995; **45** (395): 283–285.
2. Holland L. Cardiovascular medicines. *Br Hom J* 1994; **83**: 223–229.
3. Blackie M. *Classical Homoeopathy.* Beaconsfield: Beaconsfield Publishers, 1990.
4. Clarke JH. *The Prescriber*. Saffron Walden: Health Science Press, 1985.

Gastrointestinal problems

Anal fissure

Aesculus:	Dry aching, feels full of sticks. Anus raw with sharp shooting pains. Large dry hard stools. Burning in anus with chills up and down back.
Chamomilla:	Soreness of anus.
Graphites:	Smarting sore anus with itching. Fissure.
Nitric acid:	Great straining but little passes. Rectum feels torn. Tearing pain during stool. Violent pain after stool, lasting hours.
Rathania:	Aches as if full of broken glass. Burns for hours after passing stool. Anus feels constricted. Relieved temporarily by cold water.
Silica:	Fissures with spasm of rectum. Bashful stool. Faeces retained for long time.

Colic

This particularly relates to colic in children.

Bryonia:	Irritable and cross. Worse for movement. Constipation with thirst for cold drinks. Worse for warm applications.
Chamomilla:	Moans and screams with pain. Restless and irritable, relieved by nursing. Better for heat and being carried.
Colocynth:	Doubles up with pain. Restless and irritable. Better for bending, firm pressure, lying and passing wind.
Mag. phos.:	Sensitive to cold, anxious. Wind and bloating. Better for doubling up, rubbing and belching.

Constipation

It is obviously important to exclude sinister pathology when dealing with this problem. A full examination and further investigation may be necessary before treatment can begin. A list of remedies is found in Chapter 27.

Diarrhoea and vomiting

This is common syndrome in general practice, particularly if induced by food poisoning, which is definitely on the increase, or viral gastro-enteritis. Many cases respond to simple first aid advice regarding adequate hygiene measures and rehydration. Homoeopathy can sometimes ease symptoms.

Aloes:	Aversion to meat. Nausea. Constant bearing-down in rectum. Flatus. Rectum feels insecure; bearing-down sensation as if everything will come away. Burning in anus.
Arsenicum album:	Vomiting and diarrhoea after eating spoiled food. Exhaustion and prostration. Chilly, better for warmth. Burning sensation relieved by warmth and by small amounts of drinks at intervals.
Ipecac:	Tongue clean. Much saliva, constant nausea and vomiting. Frothy green stool. Sensation of need to empty bowels.
Merc. corrosivus:	Tenesmus, not relieved by passing stool. Hot, bloody and slimy. Abdomen painful to touch.
Podphyllum:	Long-standing diarrhoea early in morning. Painless. Profuse green and gushing. (POD = profuse, offensive, dawn.)

For diarrhoea before exams or performance, consider Arg. nit., Gelsemium, Lycopodium or Silica.

Dyspepsia

I have avoided labelling this as ulcer symptoms, but rather tried to describe symptom pictures for several remedies used for this condition.

Anacardium:	Weak digestion with fullness and distension. Empty feeling in stomach with nausea. Eating

relieves the dyspepsia. Swallows food and drink hastily. Sensation of a plug in various parts.

Arsenicum album: Burning in stomach relieved by small sips of cold water. Restless.

Bryonia: Nausea and faintness when rising. Thirst for large amounts. Worse for warm drinks. Sensitive stomach. Pressure after eating. Worse in summer heat.

Lycopodium: Dyspepsia due to fermentable foods, beans, cabbage, etc. Excessive hunger. Desire for sweets. Food tastes sour. Pressure in stomach after eating. Fullness after a few mouthfuls. Likes to take food hot. Bloated and full sensation.

Nux vomica: Hangover remedy. Nausea in morning after eating. Stomach sensitive to pressure. Bloated several hours after eating. Loves fats and tolerates them well. Flatulent distension.

Phosphorus: Hunger soon after eating. Belching large quantities. Vomiting water as soon as it warms in stomach. Pain relieved by cold liquids and ices.

Robinia: Dull heavy aching in stomach; acrid eructations. Colic and flatulence. Sour eructations. Distension of stomach.

Haemorrhoids

Aesculus: Venous stasis. Dry and aching; rectum feels full of sticks. Piles bleed with sharp pains up and down back.

Aloes: Piles protrude like grapes. Diarrhoea with sense of insecurity in rectum.

Hamamelis: Piles bleed profusely, soreness. Anus raw and sore. Rectum feels bruised.

Wind

This covers a variety of symptom presentations. There are several useful 'windy' remedies.

Argent nit.:	Belching, flatulence with painful swelling at pit of stomach. Craving for sweets. Burning and eructations. Colic with distension.
Carbo. veg.:	Eructations, heaviness, fullness after eating and drinking. Relief after belching. Burning pain in stomach. Pain half-hour after eating. Faint sensation in stomach not relieved by eating. Averse to milk, meat and fatty things.
China:	Flatulent colic. Flatulence, belching gives no relief.
Lycopodium:	Eating causes fullness. Incomplete burning eructations, which rise and cause burning sensation. Abdomen bloated and full.
Pulsatilla:	Averse to fatty food, warm food and drink. Tastes remain for a long time. Flatulence, dislikes butter. Thirstlessness with all complaints. Pain in stomach an hour after eating.

23

Homoeopathy for children

When considering the content of this chapter I took particular note of the views of my health visitor colleagues who produced a list of common symptoms on which they are asked to give advice. In primary care, consultations with children under the age of 15 account for about 12% of all contacts with the doctor. With this in mind, I have tried to produce a useful and logical list of treatments for common symptoms. These are discussed in Chapter 25.

Whilst it is true that many conditions are self-limiting and need only reassurance, there is a group of common complaints that responds well to homoeopathy.

When considering treatment it is reasonable to consider various approaches. Many presentations are acute and in these cases low-potency remedies given frequently may help. In chronic cases a more thorough approach is needed, with a constitutional remedy perhaps with a nosode or miasmatic treatment in a complex case.

Borland[1] produced an excellent booklet, *Childrens' Types*, in which he classified children into various groups depending on the remedy. His description of how children may progress from one remedy type to another as they grow is interesting, and readers are recommended to study this publication to help them understand remedy actions.

There are five groups:

1. The *fat, fair, chilly* and *lethargic* group:

Calc. carb.	Calc. phos.
Phos.	Silica
Sanicula	Aethusa
Lycopodium	Causticum
Tuberculinum	

2. The *delayed* and *backward* group:

Bartya carb.	Borax
Natrum mur.	Sepia
Aurum met.	Carbo. veg.

3. '*Skins*':

Graphites	Capsicum
Psorinum	Antimonium crud.
Petroleum	

4. *Warm-blooded* remedies:

Pulsatilla	Kali. sulph.
Sulphur	Thuja
Bromium	Iodum
Abronatum	Fluoricum acidum

5. The *nervy types*:

Arsenicum alb.	Chamomilla
China	Mag. carb.
Ignatia	Zincum

Herscu[2], in his book, *The Homoeopathic Treatment of Children*, concentrates on a group of eight remedies which make up 80% of his paediatric practice. The remedies, Calc. carb., Lycopodium, Medorrhinum, Natrum mur., Phosphorus, Pulsatilla, Sulphur and Tuberculinum, make an interesting list and his book comprehensively discusses specific features of these remedies in children.

References

1. Borland D. *Children's types*. London: British Homoeopathic Association, 1950.
2. Herscu P. *The Homoeopathic Treatment of Children.* Berkeley, CA: North Atlantic Books, 1991.

Section 4

Homoeopathy and the Community Health Care Team

24

Homoeopathy for the primary care nursing team

In the following chapters I will try to condense the use of remedies into specific fields that the nurse, midwife or health visitor may find they require. I have not attempted to impose my own views on this area, but have consulted with members of my team who have taken an interest and sometimes wanted to use complementary therapies.

As elsewhere, this chapter is introductory and cannot be exhaustive. The commonest conditions are listed with a range of possible remedies. Further references are available at the end of the book. Many conditions and potential treatments are discussed in other sections.

A recent survey of nurses showed that 58% of nurses[1] had used some form of complementary therapy in their work. It is perhaps not surprising that the most popular treatments were those which are easier to learn, are of daily value in a range of conditions and do not require extensive training. The most popular therapies were massage and aromatherapy.

It is reassuring that, of those who have practised some form of complementary therapy, just over 25% would like to learn more about homoeopathy.

The range of conditions for which nurses have used complementary therapies includes relaxation, stress, pain, anxiety, insomnia and pregnancy and labour. The list of conditions for which they have used complementary therapies for themselves, friends or family included stress, pain, backache, headache/migraine, anxiety, colds/flu, insomnia, arthritis, skin problems, premenstrual tension, asthma and depression. Many of these conditions are recognized to be responsive to homoeopathy.

Homoeopathy for the health visitor (see Chapter 25)

Colic
Teething
Earache
Eczema
Asthma
Colds/flu

Nappy rash
Cuts and bruises
Hayfever
Impetigo
Sticky eyes
Sleep problems

Homoeopathy for the midwife (see Chapter 26)

Premenstrual tension
Morning sickness
Pregnancy
Labour
Postoperative wound care
Post-delivery
Breast care

Homoeopathy and the district nurse (see Chapter 27)

Cystitis
Constipation
Wound pain and postoperative problems
Bruising
Cuts
Skin problems
Leg ulcers

Complementary therapies and the nursing profession

The nursing profession is undergoing continual change. The 1992 United Kingdom Central Council (UKCC) document *The Scope of Professional Practice* gave nurses guidelines to extend practice and the nurses role and responsibilities. It is my view that all practitioners using complementary therapies should have had approved training by a recognized body.

Therapies may be given in a variety of settings – self-help, first aid or practical therapeutic advice. Of course appropriate approval from nursing management is required, as well as from the doctors who retain ultimate responsibility for their patient's care.

Reference

1. Alternative update. A true complement ? *Nursing Times* 1996; **92**(5): 42–44.

25
Common childhood problems: a guide for the GP and health visitor

Homoeopathy for the health visitor

- Colic
- Teething
- Earache
- Eczema
- Asthma
- Colds/flu
- Nappy rash
- Cuts and bruises
- Hayfever
- Impetigo
- Sticky eyes
- Sleep problems

In approaching these conditions my first recommendation would be to provide reassurance and wait (see aphorism 150). Just because you know about homoeopathy does not mean that a patient always needs a remedy. Many conditions resolve spontaneously with support and encouragement. However homoeopathy is an attractive treatment to an increasingly consumer-conscious public, concerned with issues such as drug side-effects.

I make no attempt to include the treatment of complicated conditions in this book. Rather the aim is to provide an *aide-mémoire* for those who repeatedly come across the same conditions and struggle to find the correct homoeopathic remedy.

Acute remedies can be repeated frequently in children and a dose of 6C or 30C would be used. For a chronic case a single dose of a constitutional remedy may be given and not repeated too frequently. In classical homoeopathy the practitioner should wait until there is no more benefit to be gained from the single dose before repeating or changing the treatment (see Chapter 12).

Conjunctivitis

Argent nit.:	Yellow or white discharge. Pink injected whites.
Arsenicum alb.:	Burning irritation.
Calc. carb.:	Sticky lids, especially in morning. Sensitive to light.
Pulsatilla:	Profuse bland discharge. Thick yellow. Itching and burning.
Sulphur:	Burning ulceration of margins.

Colic

Chamomilla:	Sensitive, irritable, wind passed with no relief. Carrying helps. One cheek red and hot.
Colocynthus:	Rolling around, bends over for relief. Relieved by pressure. Left-sided.
Mag. phos.:	Cramping pains, better for heat and relieved by rubbing, warmth and pressure.
Nux vom.:	Chilly and irritable. Distended with colic.
Pulsatilla:	Windy and crying. Pitiful, better for comfort.

Diarrhoea

Arsenicum alb.:	Painless and watery stool. Offensive with prostration. Worse at night and after eating and drinking. Restless and thirsty.
Chamomilla:	Hot, green, watery and fetid stool. Slimy with colic, like chopped spinach. Flushed and irritable.
Ipecac:	With vomiting and nausea. Green stool.
Merc. sol.:	Hot, bloody, slimy stool with tenesmus.

Other remedies may include Aethusa, Aloes, Podophyllum and phosphorus, but a more detailed description is warranted, with reference to Materia Medica.

Nappy rash

Calc. carb.:	Chilly baby, fat and flabby. Sweaty head. Unhealthy skin does not heal easily.
Sulphur:	Hot child, worse for heat and bathing. Offensive discharges.

Earache

Aconite:	Acute onset, after chill or exposure to cold. Restless and anxious. External ear hot, painful and swollen.
Belladonna:	Throbbing, heat and redness. Flushed child, dilated pupils. Otitis media.
Chamomilla:	Restless, unbearable pain. Hot. Only calmed by carrying. Swelling and heat drive patient frantic.
Pulsatilla:	Difficult hearing, thick offensive yellow discharge. Worse for heat. Better for consolation.

For glue ear it may be worth considering Pulsatilla or Calc. carb. if the picture fits.

For persistent discharges from ears other remedies to consider would be Hepar sulph., Graphites, Mercurius sol., Pulsatilla or Sulphur.

Sore throat

Rather than labelling the throat as tonsillitis consider the throat by its appearance and symptom picture.

Aconite:	Sudden onset, after exposure to cold dry weather. Early stages of flu.
Bartya carb.:	Frequent sore throats with persistently enlarged glands in undersized children. Prone to colds, and suppurating tonsils with every sore throat. Can only swallow liquids.
Belladonna:	Dry, congested and hot. Worse on right side, tongue feels constricted. Swallowing worse for liquids. Thirstless.
Calc. carb.:	Fat, fair and chilly. Persistent enlarged cervical nodes. Swollen tonsils.

Hepar sulph.:	Chilly, sensation of a plug when swallowing. Yellow exudate. Pain extends to ears.
Merc. sol.:	Red, swollen and inflamed. Intensely inflamed. Burning pain with anxiety. Salivation. Tongue coated and yellow and indented by teeth.
Phytolacca:	Dark red or bluish. Shooting pain to ears. Grey exudate, like membrane. Cannot swallow anything hot. Swollen glands and stiff neck.
Sulphur:	Persistent sore throats between attacks in hot children.

Teething problems

Calc. carb.:	Fat, fair and chilly. Sweating on scalp. Late teething.
Chamomilla:	Angry, irritable, soothed by holding.

There are a variety of remedies depending on the state of the child, including Calc. phos., Kreosotum and Silica amongst the most prominent in Boericke's repertory[1].

Travel sickness

There are a variety of combined remedies available over-the-counter, and, whilst this is not classical homoeopathy – more like complex homoeopathy – they will suffice for first-aid purposes.

Cocculus:	Nausea from riding in cars, boats etc., or looking at a boat in motion. Faint. Aversion to food and sight and smell of food aggravates. Metallic taste.
Tabacum:	Seasickness, nausea and icy coldness. Vertigo on opening eyes. Worse for smell of tobacco. Band-like headache.
Petroleum:	Vertigo on rising. Nausea with accumulation of saliva in mouth. Headache relieved by pressure.

Bedwetting

This is a difficult problem which requires medical assessment, exclusion of urinary tract infection and a behavioural approach. There are many remedies in the repertory; a few common ones are mentioned below.

Causticum:	Involuntary passage of urine during first sleep at night or from excitement. Involuntary when sneezing.
Equisetum:	Incontinence with dreams and nightmares. Can have loin pain. Burning and cutting in urethra may occur.

Other remedies mentioned in Boericke[1] are Gelsemium, Kreosotum, Nux vom., Sepia and Sulphur.

Sleep problems

Aconite:	Restlessness and excitement. Nightmares and anxious dreams. Long dreams.
Argentum nit.:	Anticipatory anxiety leading to restlessness and poor sleep.
Arnica:	Unable to sleep despite being tired. Bed feels hard.
Coffea cruda:	Wakeful, constantly moving about. Wakes at 3 a.m., sleep disturbed by dreams. Mental activity, flow of ideas.
Ignatia:	Very light sleep, jerkiness of limbs. Worries prevent sleep.
Nux vom.:	Cannot sleep after 3 a.m. until morning. May have dyspepsia. Wakes feeling awful. Dreams full of activity, better for short naps.

Colds and flu (see pp. 71–72)

In the early stages Aconite is recommended; this may be followed by Arsenicum alb., Euphrasia, Allium cepa or Ferr. phos. and Gelsemium, depending on the symptom picture. As a cold develops then other remedies may be needed.

Bryonia:	Sore throat, cough, irritable and dry mucous membranes. Thirst. Worse for movement, better for rest. Right sided chest symptoms.

Ferrum phos.:	Between aconite and belladonna. Nervous sensitive with facial flushing. Prostration. Short painful tickling cough. Hoarseness.
Gelsemium:	Dull, heavy-eyed. Aches and pains in limbs and back. Headache relieved by passing urine. Exertion causes fatigue and muscle trembling.

Infectious diseases of childhood

Measles

In the early stages remedies such as Aconite may be useful, but when the condition progresses the following may be of help.

Belladonna:	Hot, restless and irritable. Red face. Flushed and throbbing headaches. Thirstless.
Euphrasia:	For conjunctival symptoms.
Pulsatilla:	Tired, restless and whimpering. Profuse catarrhal discharges. Better for cool air.
Sulphur:	Dusky rash, hot. Worse for heat and at night.
Morbillinum:	For prevention or after-effect of acute disease.

Chickenpox

Antimonium tart.:	Pustular eruption leaving bluish-red mark.
Ranunculus:	Burning and intense itching. Pustules, especially thoracic shingles. Bluish pustules.
Rhus tox.:	Red and swollen with intense itching. Restlessness.

Pratt[2] suggests a regime of Aconite in the early stages, Rhus tox. when the blisters form, Merc. sol. during convalescence and Varicellinum when there are prolonged after-effects.

Pertussis

Pertussin:	This is claimed to have a protective effect if there is a local outbreak, or to follow an attack if there are prolonged symptoms.
Antimonium tart.:	Cough with rattling of mucus, but little expectorated. Burning spreads to throat, better lying on right.

Cuprum met.:	Suffocative attacks, worse at 3 a.m. Spasm and constriction. Better for drinking cold water.
Drosera:	Cough, worse after midnight. Spasmodic, paroxysms. Hoarseness. Choking sensation.
Hepar sulph.:	Chilly. Cough whenever body exposed to cold. Choking cough. Suffocative attacks.
Ipecac:	Constriction of chest, incessant and violent cough. Nose bleed associated. Nausea.

Glandular fever

This is still a common condition. I treat early phases as for sore throat or colds depending on symptoms. For post-viral malaise I use the glandular fever nosode or carcinosin.

Reference

1. Boericke W. *Pocket Manual of Homoeopathic Materia Medica* (ninth edn). New Delhi: B Jain Publishers, 1988.
2. Pratt N. *Homoeopathic Prescribing*. Beaconsfield: Beaconsfield Publishers, 1985.

Homoeopathy in pregnancy: Remedies for the GP and midwife

Homoeopathy for the midwife

- Premenstrual tension
- Morning sickness
- Pregnancy
- Labour
- Postoperative wound care
- Post-delivery
- Breast care

The nursing profession is taking a great interest in the use of complementary medicine. This is confirmed by the increasing number of courses in the various therapies. Homoeopathy rates highly amongst the therapies; particularly so in pregnancy because of its safety and lack of effect on the fetus.

This chapter covers the common problems encountered by GPs and midwives.

I reiterate that there is absolutely no substitute for sound clinical practice. However homoeopathy provides a gentle approach to the management of many problems seen in practice.

Morning sickness

Ipecac:	Constant nausea not relieved by vomiting. Clean tongue, much saliva. Pallor. Vomits food, bile and mucus. Stomach feels relaxed. Irritable.
Kreosotum:	Nausea, vomiting of food several hours after eating. Feeling of ice-cold water in stomach.

Nux vom.:	Nausea in morning. Worse for eating. Nausea and vomiting with retching. Worse in morning. Chilly and irritable.
Sepia:	Empty feeling not relieved by eating. Nausea at smell or sight of food. Nausea in morning. Desires pickles, acids and vinegar. Worse after milk and loathes fat.

Other remedies include Apomorph, Arsenicum, Cimcifuga and Pulsatilla.

Leg cramps

This is sometimes an irritating symptom in pregnancy. Allopathic remedies are contraindicated.

Cuprum met.:	Jerking, twitching of muscles. Cold hands. Cramps in calves and soles.
Nux vom.:	Legs numb, cramps in calves and soles.

Back pain (see Chapter 17)

Breast problems

Sore nipples

Chamomilla:	Inflamed and tender. Painful with cracks and fissures. Mother irritable. (Cream also used).

Breast pain

Belladonna:	For areas of hot, tender and painful breasts with throbbing pain.
Conium:	Breasts hard and painful to touch. Stitches in nipples.
Phytolacca:	Mastitis. Breasts hard and very tender. Mammary abscess. Pain radiates from nipple all over breast when feeding. Cracks and small ulcers around nipples.

Pre- and post-delivery

Studies have demonstrated the benefits of homoeopathic treatment before and during labour. My own experience in this area is limited, but the remedies are mentioned and references given.

Labour pain

Braxton Hicks type

Caulophyllum: False labour pain. Colicky lower abdominal pain.

Cimcifuga: Pain across pelvis from hip to hip. Pre- and post-labour contractions.

Before labour

Consider advising the use of any of the following before labour.

Arnica: To reduce bruising and bleeding.

Hypericum: To reduce the pain from tissue damage in the perineum.

Labour

There is some evidence for the use of homoeopathy in labour to promote uterine contractions. Remedies of particular value include caulophyllum and Pulsatilla, Arnica, Secale and Cimcifuga (actaea racemosa). An interesting and thorough review of this subject is given by Moskowitz[1].

After labour

Arnica: Sore, bruised, aches all over.

Causticum: With urinary symptoms or irritation to bladder. Unable to pass urine.

Hypericum: For sensitive tissue damage in perineum either from tear or episiotomy.

Staphysagria: Used for urinary symptoms, but also useful for post hysterectomy wound pain.

Postnatally

Many of the above remedies are useful for the problems associated with delivery. Two useful pregnancy remedies which should be studied in more detail are Caulophyllum and Cimcifuga. Both have an effect on uterine contraction but, whilst caulophyllum is predominantly useful in this area, both during pregnancy and for a variety of problems associated with painful menses, Cimcifuga (actaea racemosa) is associated with strong mental symptoms.[2]

Cimcifuga is useful in neuralgias but its mental symptoms, particularly postnatally are strong. The patient feels morose and dejected, with negative feelings. She has a sense of a black cloud hanging over her. She fears something terrible is going to happen and there is a strong feeling of insanity.

Reference

1. Moskowitz R. *Homoeopathic Medicines in Pregnancy and Childbirth*. Berkeley, CA: North Atlantic Books, 1992.
2. Moskowitz R. Two childbirth remedies. *Br Hom J* 1990; **79**: 206–211.

27

Homoeopathy and the district nurse

Homoeopathy and the district nurse

- Cystitis
- Constipation
- Wound pain and postoperative problems
- Bruising
- Cuts
- Skin problems
- Leg ulcers

In this chapter only those conditions described by my team of nurses as occurring frequently are included.

Cystitis (see Chapter 20)

Urinary incontinence

It is important to exclude urinary tract infection, constipation, pelvic masses and prostatic problems in these patients.

Apis mel:	Frequent and involuntary voiding. Burning and soreness. Strangury. Last drop burns and stings.
Belladonna:	Sensitive in bladder region. Incontinence with continuous dropping. Frequent and profuse passage of urine. Prostatic hypertrophy.
Benzoic acid:	Repulsive odour, enuresis and dribbling in old men.
Causticum:	Involuntary when coughing or sneezing.

	Expelled slowly. Involuntary passage at night or from slight excitement.
Equisetum:	Frequent urging with severe pain at the close of urination. Urine flows drop by drop. Burning and cutting pain in urethra.
Pulsatilla:	Increased desire, especially when lying down. Involuntary micturition at night, when coughing or passing flatus.

Constipation

Aesculus (chestnut):	Dry aching rectum, feels full of sticks. Pain after stool. Large, hard, dry stool with burning in anus and chills up and down back.
Alumen: (common potash)	Constipation of severest form. No desire for stool, with ineffectual urging. No ability to expel stool. Marble-like stool passes, but rectum still feels full. Long-lasting pain and smarting after stool.
Alumina:	Hard, dry, knotty stool. No desire to pass. Straining. Evacuation preceded by painful urging long before stool, then straining at stool.
Bryonia:	Dry, hard, knotty stool. Worse in morning and from moving.
Calc. carb.:	Crawling and constriction of rectum. Large and hard stool.
Hydrastis:	Constipation with sinking feeling in stomach, and dull headache. After stool, long-lasting pain.
Lycopodium:	Stool hard, ineffectual, small and incomplete.
Nitric acid:	Great straining but little passes. Constipated with anal fissures. Tearing pain during stool. Pain lasts hours after stool.
Nux vomica:	Constipation with ineffectual urging. Feeling that some remains unexpelled. Passes small quantities each time. Alternate constipation and diarrhoea.
Opium:	Obstinate constipation. No desire to pass stool. Round, hard, black balls. Faeces protrude then recede. (Thuja and silica.) Violent pain in rectum.

Sepia: Constipation with large, hard stools and feeling as if there is a ball in the rectum. Tenesmus with pains shooting upwards. Bearing-down sensation.

Postoperative and wound care

Arnica: Pain, bruising and swelling.

Calendula: Either as tincture applied locally or taken internally for grazes and wounds that will not heal. Promotes epithelialization.

Cantharis: For burns and scalds.

Hepar sulph.: Infected wounds. Chilly, sensitive to cold and air.

Hypericum: For injuries to nerves. Pain after operations. Lacerated wounds with prostration due to blood loss.

Phosphorus: Wounds that bleed easily even if small, then heal and break out again. Purpura and ecchymoses.

Silica: Abscesses and old fistulous ulcers which fail to heal. Promotes expulsion of foreign bodies. Every little injury suppurates. Keloid growths.

Thiosinnamium: (oil of mustard seed) Dissolves scar tissue.

Staphysagria: Sensitive, good for pain after incised wounds.

Symphytum: Good for stimulating periosteal growth, after fractures.

Leg ulcers and skin care

The great variety of treatments is testimony to the problem of venous ulceration in the community. The time and expense spent on this condition are phenomenal. The basic tenets of good care are rest, elevation and compression. Attention must be paid to nutrition and tissue viability, excluding other underlying causes if possible, like varicose veins, vasculitis or arterial insufficiency.

Belladonna: Hot, red, swollen suppurative wounds. Redness of skin. Chronic induration after inflammation.

Calendula: Useful for open wounds applied topically as dilute tincture, cream or internally. Promotes

	granulation; useful on burns and scalds and erysipelas.
Hamamelis:	Bluish lesions, phlebitis and purpura. Varicose veins and ulcers which are very sore.
Hydrastis:	Ulcers with thick yellow ropy discharge.
Kali. bich.:	Ulcers with punched-out edges, penetrating and thick exudate. Migrating pains.
Nitric acid:	Ulcers which bleed easily with splinter-like pains and irregular edges. Base looks like raw flesh.
Phosphorus:	Small ulcers which bleed easily.
Silica:	Indurated slow-healing lesions.
Syphilinum:	Reddish brown skin eruption. Recurrent abscesses and widespread ulceration associated with rheumatic pains. Pains worse at night.

Varicose veins

It is best to prevent venous ulcers by treating of the underlying varicose veins by surgery. The following remedies may be of use for problems with the veins themselves .

Arnica:	Veins swollen and feel bruised after trauma.
Fluoric acid:	Particularly good for varicose veins and associated ulcers which have red edges. Worse for warmth.
Hamamelis:	Very sore veins, bruised sensation, much venous congestion. Useful for open wounds with weakness from blood loss and with venous oozing.

Topical applications

Although Hahnemann was damning about the use of topical preparations, which he felt masked signs of underlying internal conditions, there are a variety of useful topical agents. These are available as unpotentized tinctures, which may be diluted in water or mixed with cream, such as Arnica, Calendula, Hypercal (mixture of hypericum and calendula). Alternatively, genuine potentized preparations of remedies in a cream or ointment base include Arnica, Calendula, Graphites, Hamamelis, Hypericum, Paeonia, Rhus tox., Tamus and Urtica urens.

Section 5

Materia Medica

Materia medica – a guide

No materia medica in this format can be exhaustive. I have tried to include remedies with everyday uses which are mentioned in the Primary Care Certificate courses and added a few remedies which I use frequently in practice.

Knowing the remedies enables you to use them regularly without complex repertorization. Symptom pictures and keynotes become familiar with use and some trial and error may be necessary.

Each patient should be thoroughly assessed; and homoeopathy cannot replace the fundamentals of good clinical practice.

Aconite

Source	Monkshood.
Uses	States of anxiety, mental restlessness. Acute illnesses. Brief duration of action.
Mind	Fear, anxiety with every ailment. Forebodings, fears death. Fears the future, fears crowds, fears crossing the street. Restlessness. Intolerable pains.
Head	Heavy, hot bursting headache. Vertigo, worse on rising.
Eyes	Dry and hot. Watering after exposure to dry cold winds.
Nose	Acute sense of smell. Pain at root of nose. Dry blocked nose.
Face	Red, hot, flushed and swollen. One cheek red, the other pale. Left-sided neuralgia.
Throat	Red, dry and constricted.
Stomach	Vomiting with fear.
Respiratory	Dry, coarse, croupy cough. Worse after midnight.
Heart	Palpitations after neuralgia.

Extremities	Hot hands and cold feet. Numbness and tingling.
Fever	Cold chills. Thirst with restlessness.
Modalities	< warm room < at night < dry cold winds <music < tobacco smoke > open air

Keynotes

Fear and anxiety.
Dry hot skin.
Restlessness.
Worse for dry cold winds.
Croup.

Apis mellifica

Source	The honey bee (whole insect)
Uses	Bites, stings, urticaria. Oedema. Constricted sensations. Effusions and inflammations.
Mind	Apathy, jealous, tearfulness. Listless.
Head	Brain feels tired. Throbbing pains > pressure < motion.
Eyes	Swollen, red, oedematous lids. Lacrimation hot. Exudation and suppuration. Styes.
Mouth	Red, swollen, like erysipelas. Tongue fiery, red, swollen and sore.
Urine	Scant. Burns.
Extremities	Oedema. Swollen, shiny joints with stinging pain.
Skin	Swellings after bites. Sore, sensitive.
Fever	With thirst.
Modalities	< heat < touch < pressure < right side. > open air > cold bathing.

Keynotes

Burning, stinging sore.
Oedema with redness. Relief from cold applications.
Fever with thirst.

Argentum nitricum

Source	Nitrate of silver
Uses	Good for neuroses, anticipatory anxiety. Effects of prolonged mental exertion.
Mentals	Fearful and nervous. Melancholic. Time passes slowly. Impulsive. Anticipatory anxiety.
Head	Hemicranial headaches. > pressure < mental exertion.
Eyes	Purulent conjunctivitis. Swelling of conjunctiva.
Face	Sunken, pale, tight drawing of skin over bones.
Throat	Sensation of splinter in throat on swallowing.
Stomach	Belching. Gnawing ulcer pain. Craving for sweets.
Extremities	Trembling with debility.
Modalites	< warmth, at night, cold food < sweets < after food > eructation, fresh air, cold, pressure.

Keynotes

Anticipatory anxiety with diarrhoea.
Chilly, yet feels smothered if wrapped up.
Conjunctivitis.
Belching with gastric ailments.
Sensation of splinter in throat.

Arnica

Source	Plant: leopard's bane.
Uses	When injury of any type may have caused symptoms.
Mind	Indifference. Denies there is anything wrong. Wants to be left alone.
Head	Hot head, cold body. Effects of trauma to head.
Eyes	Feels tired after excess use. Bruised feeling after close work.
Female	Bruised parts after labour.
Heart	Angina. Left arm.
Skin	Black and blue. Bruising.
Sleep	Restless when overtired.
Modalities	< touch, motion, rest. > lying down or with head low.

Keynotes

Sore lame feeling throughout body as if beaten.
Whenever lie down the surface seems too hard.
Traumatic injuries.
Nervous, cannot endure pain.

Arsenicum album

Source	White oxide of arsenic.
Uses	Diarrhoea and vomiting. Neuroses.
Mind	Prostration, anxiety, fearful and restless. Mentally restless. Fear of death and ill health. Irritable.
Head	Headache relieved by cold, other symptoms better for heat.
Eyes	Burning with lacrimation. Photophobia.
Nose	Thin excoriating discharge.
Throat	Burning, swollen and oedematous.
Stomach	Cannot bear sight or smell of food. Great thirst. Drinks much but little at a time. Burning pain in stomach. Craves acid and coffee.
Stool	Small, offensive and dark with prostration. Worse at night and after eating and drinking. Burning pain in anus.
Female	Menorrhagia.
Respiratory	Fears suffocation. Asthma worse at night. Frothy expectoration.
Heart	Palpitations
Skin	Itching, burning. Oedema. Dry, rough, scaly, worse in cold. Ulcers, offensive discharge. Psoriasis.
Modalities	< wet weather < after midnight < cold. > heat, warm drinks, elevated.

Keynotes

Burning pains, prostration, restlessness.
Chilly, better for heat.
Fears suffocation, death, ill health.

Belladonna

Source	Plant: deadly nightshade.
Uses	Nervous excitement, violent throbbing pain with heat and redness.
Mind	Hallucinations, rages, delirium (c.f. Hyoscyanamus, Stramonium.)
Head	Vertigo, falling to left or backwards. Throbbing and heat. Pain, especially forehead. Worse for noise, movement and lying down, better for pressure and semierect.
Face	Red, hot swollen.
Eyes	Dilated pupils.
Ears	Middle-ear pain. Otitis media. Throbbing.
Throat	Dry, red and angry. Worse on right.
Stomach	Thirst for cold water.
Abdomen	Distended, hot.
Female	Forcing downwards of genitals. Bright red and profuse haemorrhage. Mastitis, hot and throbbing breast.
Heart	Palpitations, throbbing all through the body.
Skin	Dry, red, swollen and hot. Boils, rosacea. Fever. No thirst with fever.
Modalities	< touch, draught, lying down, afternoon. > semi-erect.

Keynotes

Heat.
Redness.
Throbbing.

Bryonia

Source	Wild hops.
Uses	Coughs, colds, influenza. Ailments with characteristic pains.
Mind	Irritable. Bad tempered.
Head	Bursting, splitting headache. Worse from motion, stooping and opening eyes.

Eyes	Pressing pain.
Mouth	Lips parched, dry and cracked. Dry mouth and excessive thirst.
Stomach	Pressure in stomach after eating. Liver region sore, burning pain.
Stool	Constipation; dry, hard stool. Worse in morning.
Respiratory	Dry cough. Stitches in chest. Worse on entering a warm room.
Joints	Hot, red and swollen. Worse for least movement.
Modalities	< warmth < motion < morning and after eating < hot weather. > lying on affected side > pressure > rest > cold.

Keynotes

Irritable.
Dry.
Worse for motion.
Better for rest.
Right-sided.
Thirst (large quantities at long intervals).

Calc. carb.

Source	Middle layer of oyster shell.
Uses	Consititutional remedy. Impaired nutrition affecting skin, glands and bone. Antipsoric.
Mind	Fears. Likes routine. Forgetful. Adverse to work and mental exertion.
Head	Vertigo on ascending. Icy coldness of head. Profuse perspiration. Enlarged head in children. Sweats.
Ears	Chronic purulent discharge and enlarged glands.
Nose	Nasal polypi. Colds with each change of weather.
Face	Pale with dark rings around eyes.
Throat	Swelling of tonsils. Goitre.
Stomach	Aversion to meat. Craves indigestible things like chalk and coal. Likes eggs, salt and sweets. Dislikes fats. Desires long cold drinks.

Abdomen	Distension. Cannot bear tight clothing around waist.
Female	Profuse early menses. Leukorrhoea. Breasts tender and swollen before menses.
Respiratory	Cough, worse at night. Painless hoarseness. Tightness, burning going up stairs. Desires fresh air.
Extremeties	Rheumatic pains after exposure to wet weather (chronic of rhus tox.). Cold damp feet. Raw soles of feet.
Skin	Unhealthy, flaccid skin. Swollen glands. Eczema.
Modalities	< exertion < cold < wet weather. > dry climate > lying on painful side.

Keynotes

Fat and flabby.
Chilly, dislikes cold.
Head sweats profusely while sleeping.
Fleshy and grows too rapidly.
Disease due to ossification delay.
Slow to walk or stand.
Coldness of single parts.

Calendula

Source	Marigold.
Uses	Healing agent both internally and externally.
Mind	Nervous, frightened.
Eyes	Tendency to suppuration.
Skin	For sloughy wounds. Superficial burns and scalds.
Modalities	< damp, heavy, cloudy weather.

Use as cream, diluted tincture or internally.

Cantharis

Source	Spanish fly (crushed and potentized).
Uses	Principally urinary organs.
Mind	Delirium. Restless, acute mania.
Head	Burning pains.

Throat	Covered in vesicles. Burning of mucous membranes. Aphthous ulcers. Difficulty swallowing liquids.
Stomach	Violent burning. Disgust for food.
Urine	Intolerable urging. Raw burning pains with constant desire to pass urine. Urine scalds and is passed drop by drop. Urine jelly-like and shreddy.
Male	Increased libido.
Female	Nymphomania. Burning in pelvis.
Skin	Vesicular eruptions, burning and itching. Burns and scalds relieved by cold. Erysipelas.
Modalities	< touch, urinating.

Keynotes

Burning in all parts.
Urging to urinate.
Increased sexual desire.

Carbo. veg.

Source	Vegetable charcoal.
Uses	Chronic complaints in sluggish fat types. Patient is blue, has poor circulation, collapses. Slow recovery from other illnesses.
Mind	Averse to dark.
Head	Ache from overindulgence.
Face	Puffy, cyanotic. Cold sweat.
Stomach	Eructations and heaviness after eating. Distension of abdomen. Faint, empty sensation not relieved by eating. Averse to milk, meat and fats.
Stool	Corrosive discharge.
Respiratory	Cough with burning in chest.
Skin	Cold, blue. Ecchymoses. Moist skin. Varicose ulcers.
Modalities	< evening < open air < cold. > eructations > from fanning.

Keynotes

Cold with cold sweat.
Desire to be constantly fanned.
Simplest food disagrees.

Chamomilla

Source	German chamomile.
Uses	Mental and emotional states. Especially children.
Mind	Sensitive, irritable, thirsty and hot. Unbearable pains. Whining and restless. Child only calmed by carrying about. Impatient. Complaints from anger.
Ears	Earache driving child frantic.
Face	One cheek hot, the other pale and cold. Toothache, worse after warm drinks.
Abdomen	Flatulent colic after anger. Green slimy stool.
Modalities	< heat, anger, wind. > being carried, wet weather.

Keynotes

Irritable.
Quiet only when carried.
Ailments after anger.
Unendurable pain.
Offensive stool.

Cocculus

Source	Indian cockle.
Uses	Specific conditions.
Mind	Time passes quickly. Profound sadness. Anxious about health of others. Bad effect of loss of sleep.
Head	Vertigo on riding or sitting up, or even looking at a boat in motion. Headache in occiput.
Face	Facial nerve paralysis.
Stomach	Nausea from riding in cars. Aversion to taste. Metallic taste in mouth. Smell of food disgusts.

Menses	Weakness during menses, unable to stand.
Extremeties	Trembling and pain in limbs.
Modalities	< motion < loss of sleep < menses.

Keynotes

Nausea and vomiting from riding and motion.
Bad effects of loss of sleep.
Weakness during menses.

Colocynth

Source	Bitter cucumber.
Uses	Head and abdominal symptoms. Neuralgias. Cramp.
Head	Vertigo when turning to left. Pain and soreness of scalp. Burning and tearing pain.
Eyes	Sharp boring pain, better for pressure.
Face	Tearing and shooting pain of face. Left-sided soreness. Relief from pressure.
Abdomen	Agonizing, cutting pain causing patient to bend double. Worse after anger.
Female	Boring pain in ovary. Patient draws up double to relieve the pain.
Extremities	Contraction of muscles. Cramp-like pain in hip. Stiffness of joints and shortening of tendons. Better pressure and heat. Sciatic pain in left side.
Modalities	< anger and indignation. > doubling up > hard pressure > warmth.

Keynotes

Agonizing pain.
Relief from pressure.
Relief from bending double.
Left-sided facial neuralgia.

Cuprum met.

Source	Copper.
Uses	Spasmodic affections and cramps.
Mind	Mental and physical exhaustion, loss of sleep from overexertion of mind. Delirium and confusion.
Head	Convulsions. Bruised pain in eyes and brain on turning. Sense of water being poured on head.
Mouth	Strong metallic taste. Protrusion and retraction of tongue. Stammering speech.
Stomach	Nausea and vomiting, relieved by cold drink. Craves cool drink.
Abdomen	Contracted. Colic, violent and intermittent.
Stool	Painful and profuse. Cholera remedy.
Heart	Angina pectoris.
Respiratory	Cough, better for cold water. Suffocating attacks at 3 a.m. Spasm and constriction of chest. Whooping cough.
Extremeties	Jerking twitching of muscles. Cramps in calves and toes.
Modalities	< before menses. > during perspiration > drinking cold water.

Keynotes

Violent spasms and cramps.
Symptoms relieved by cold drink.

Euphrasia

Source	Eyebright.
Uses	Conjunctival inflammation producing lacrimation.
Head	Catarrhal headache.
Eyes	Catarrhal conjunctivitis. Water all the time. Acrid lacrimation, bland discharge.
Female	Amenorrhoea with ophthalmia.

Male	Prostatitis.
Modalites	< evening < indoors < light. > coffee > dark.

Keynotes

Acrid lacrimation.
Bland coryza – reverse of allium cepa.
Eyes water all the time.

Ferrum phos.

Source	Phosphate of iron.
Uses	Early febrile contractions, between aconite, belladonna and gelsemium. Pale anaemic subjects. Susceptibility to chest troubles.
Head	Sore to touch. Throbbing sensation. Headache better for cold applications. False plethora.
Nose	Predisposition to colds. Epistaxis.
Throat	Hot, red fauces. Ulcerated throat.
Stomach	Aversion to meat and milk. Vomits undigested food.
Urine	Stress incontinence.
Respiratory	First stage of all inflammatory infections. Haemoptysis. Hoarseness. Hard dry cough.
Extremeties	Rheumatism.
Modalities	< night and 4–6 p.m. < touch < motion < right side. > cold applications.

Keynotes

Nervous, sensitive, anaemic.
Susceptibility to colds and chest trouble.

Gelsemium

Source	Yellow jasmine.
Uses	Paralysis, muscular weakness, trembling. Influenza.
Mind	Dull, listless. Desires to be left alone. Apathetic about illness. Emotional excitement leading to physical symptoms. Anticipatory anxiety. Stage fright.
Head	Vertigo spreading from occiput. Band around head. Dull heavy ache, with heaviness of eyelids and bruised sensation. Headache preceded by blindness.
Eyes	Ptosis. Eyes heavy. Blurring in eyes. Orbital neuralgia with contraction and twitching of muscles.
Face	Hot, heavy and flushed. Dusky hue of face.
Throat	Difficulty swallowing, especially warm food. Throat rough and burning. Lump in throat cannot be swallowed. Pain from throat to ear.
Stomach	Thirstless.
Stool	Diarrhoea from emotional excitement.
Urine	Profuse, clear and watery.
Heart	Feeling of need to keep moving or heart would stop. Palpitations. Pulse weak and slow.
Back	Muscles feel bruised. Pain in muscles of neck, back and hips. Slight exertion causes fatigue.
Extremities	Cramp. Muscles weak and trembling.
Fever	Nervous chills.
Skin	Measles-like eruption.
Modalities	< damp < before thunderstorm < emotion, excitement or bad news < thinking about ailments > bending forward > profuse urination > open air.

Keynotes

Weakness and trembling.
Vertigo spreading from occiput.
Lack of muscular coordination.
Chill without thirst, running up and down the back.

Graphites

Source	Black lead.
Uses	Skin conditions (antipsoric). Tend to be fat and chilly.
Mind	Timid, cautious, indecisive. 'What pulsatilla is at menses, graphites is at climacteric'. Music makes them weep.
Head	Cobweb sensation on face. Itching eruption on face.
Eyes	Eyelids red and swollen. Eczema of lids.
Ears	Dryness of inner ear. Moisture and eruptions behind ears. Hears better in a noise.
Face	Eczema, erysipelas. Burning and stinging.
Stomach	Averse to meat. Dislikes hot drinks. Constrictive pain in stomach. Burning in stomach causes hunger. Flatulence. Stomach pain temporarily relieved by eating and hot drinks.
Abdomen	Distended abdomen, must loosen clothing.
Stool	Constipation.
Menses	Too late. Leukorrhoea, pale, profuse, white and excoriating.
Extremities	Nails thick, black and rough. Deformed and brittle.
Skin	Rough, hard and dry. Eruptions ooze a sticky yellow liquid. Unhealthy skin, every injury suppurates.
Modalities	< warmth < at night. > in dark > for wrapping up.

Keynotes

Music makes them weep.
Leukorrhoea in gushes.
Unhealthy skin, yellow sticky fluid.
Fat and chilly.
Sensitive to touch.

Hamamelis

Source	Witch hazel.
Uses	Cases of venous congestion. Piles, varicose veins.
Eyes	Cases of intraocular haemorrhage.
Nose	Profuse bleeding from nose.
Stool	Anus raw. Haemorrhoids bleeding profusely with soreness.
Female	Menses dark and profuse with soreness. Intermenstrual bleeds.
Skin	Bluish chilblains. Phlebitis. Purpura and ecchymoses. Varicose veins sore.
Modalities	< warm, moist air.

Keynotes

Bruised soreness of affected parts.
Venous congestion.

Hepar sulph.

Source	Calcium sulphide (extract of flowers of sulphur and crushed oyster shell).
Uses	Glandular conditions. Sensitive to impression. Tendency to suppuration.
Mind	Oversensitive, physically and mentally. Irritable. Anxious and sad.
Eyes	Ulcers on corneas. Eyes and lids red and inflamed.
Ears	Fetid discharge from ears.
Nose	Sore and ulcers. Thick offensive discharge. Hay fever.
Face	Yellow complexion. Lower lip cracked.
Throat	Sensation of plug or splinter in throat.
Stomach	Craves acids, wine and strong-tasting food. Averse to fats.
Abdomen	Chronic abdominal problems. Distension. Liver problems.
Male	Herpes. Genital ulcers. Itching.
Female	Abscesses of labia. Offensive leukorrhoea. Sensitive.

Respiratory	Hoarseness with loss of voice. Cough whenever any part of body becomes cold, or from eating cold food. Croup. Asthma worse in dry cold, better in damp.
Skin	Abscesses. Glands. Unhealthy skin. Chapped, cracked hands and feet. Ulcers sensitive to contact and cold. Putrid ulcers. Recurrent urticaria. Needs to be wrapped up.
Modalities	< dry cold winds < cool air < draught. > damp weather > wrapping up > warmth.

Keynotes

Slight injury causes suppuration.
Sensitive to cold.
Croupy choking cough.

Hypericum

Source	St John's wort
Uses	Crush injuries, especially to digits. Puncture wounds. Rectal pain. Coccydynia.
Rectum	Haemorrhoids with pain and bleeding.
Back	Pressure in nape of neck. Coccygeal pain from fall. Jerking and twitching of muscles.
Extremities	Crawling in hands and feet. Neuritis. Traumatic neuralgia. Crush injuries to digits.
Skin	Lacerated wounds with much blood loss.
Modalities	< cold < damp < least exposure < touch. > bending head backward.

Keynotes

Injury to parts rich in nerve endings.
Puncture wounds.

Ignatia

Source	St Ignatius bean.
Uses	Emotional states, hysteria, grief, particularly in women.
Mind	Changeable mood, introspective. Melancholic. Sighing and sobbing. Worse after shock.
Head	Hollow sensation, worse on stooping. As if a nail has been driven through the side. Congestive headaches after anger or grief. Worse after smoking.
Mouth	Toothache. Worse after drinking coffee.
Throat	Feeling as if there is a lump in throat. Globus hystericus. Stitching pain between swallowing. Extends to ear.
Stomach	All-gone feeling in stomach. Craves indigestible substances, sometimes sour things.
Rectum	Itching and stitching in rectum. Painful contractions after stool, deep in anus. Pressure as if instrument from within outwards.
Respiratory	Dry spasmodic cough. Sighing.
Female	Menses, black profuse irregular. Spasmodic pains in stomach.
Extremities	Jerking of limbs.
Modalites	< morning < open air < after meals and coffee < external warmth. > while eating > change of position.

Keynotes

Contradictory symptoms.
Moody.
Long concentrated grief.
Easily offended.
Tobacco upsets.

Kali. bich.

Source	Bichromate of potash, obtained from chromium iron ore.
Uses	Affinity with the mucous membranes; also affects urinary organs.
Head	Aching and fullness of glabella. Frontal pain, semi-lateral. Blurred vision precedes attack; relieved by lying down.
Eyes	Lids burn. Yellow ropy discharge.
Nose	Snuffles in fat, chubby babies. Pressure and pain at root of nose. Ulcerated septum. Thick discharge. Tough elastic plugs. Coryza with obstruction of nose.
Stomach	Gastritis. Round ulcer of stomach. Cannot digest meat. Desire for beer and acids.
Stool	Jelly-like, worse in mornings.
Urinary	Burning in urethra. Mucus in urine. Nephritis.
Male	Ulcers of penis.
Female	Pruritus vulvae. Burning.
Respiratory	Hoarse voice. Profuse yellow expectoration. Thick and sticky.
Extremities	Pains fly rapidly from one place to another. Worse for cold. Tearing pains in tibia.
Skin	Acne. Ulcers with punched-out edges.
Modalities	> heat < beer < morning < hot weather

Keynotes

Tough stringy mucus, drawn into strings.
Fat, light-haired.
Rheumatism alternates with gastric symptoms.
Pains in small spots, shift rapidly.

Kali. carb.

Source	Potassium carbonate.
Uses	Diseases of old people, weakness and paralysis. Tendency to obesity.
Mind	Despondent, alternating moods and irritable. Hypersensitive to pain. Dislikes being left alone.
Head	Vertigo on turning. Dryness of hair.
Eyes	Swelling over upper lids, like bags.
Nose	Stuffy in warm room. Thick yellow discharge.
Stomach	Flatulence. Desires sweets. Anxiety felt in stomach.
Rectum	Large difficult stool, with stitching pain before passage. Painful swollen haemorrhoids. Burning in rectum and anus.
Urine	Involuntary urination before coughing and sneezing.
Female	Menses early and profuse or late and scanty. Backache radiates to buttocks.
Respiratory	Pain in chest. Cutting or stitching. Worse on lying on right side. Hoarse. Cough at 3 a.m. Leaning forward relieves symptoms. Wheezing. Better in warm climate.
Heart	Weak, rapid pulse. Palpitations.
Back	Weakness in small of back. Backache during pregnancy and parturition.
Extremities	Back and legs give out. Tearing pains in limbs with swelling. Limbs tire easily.
Modalities	< after coition < cold weather < at 3 a.m. > warm weather > daytime > moving about

Keynotes

Pains – stitching, darting.
Cannot bear to be touched.
Bag-like swellings above eyes.
Backache.
Feels weak a week before menses.
Asthma 3 a.m.

Lachesis

Source	Venom of bushmaster snake (first described by Hering).
Uses	Haemorrhagic tendencies. Climacteric symptoms.
Mind	Loquacious. Restless, wants to move about. Jealous. Mentally better at night. Suspicious. Derangement of time. Religious insanity.
Head	Headache with flickering vision. Relieved by onset of menses.
Face	Left-sided neuralgia. Purple mottled appearance.
Mouth	Gums spongy and sore.
Throat	Sore. Worse on left side and swallowing liquids. Quinsy. Worse for pressure or touch or hot drinks. Purple appearance of throat. Cannot bear tight things around throat.
Stomach	Gnawing pain better for eating. Craves alcohol and oysters.
Abdomen	Cannot bear anything tight around waist.
Female	Climacteric problems. Palpitations, flashes of heat. Menses short and feeble, relieved by flow.
Respiratory	Throat sensitive to touch. Sense of suffocation. Spasm of glottis. Needs to take deep breath.
Heart	Palpitations. Constricted feeling in chest.
Back	Neuralgia of coccyx.
Skin	Hot, purplish, bluish appearance. Boils and ulcers with purple and black edges. Purpura. Varicose ulcers.
Modalities	< after sleep lachesis sleeps into aggravation. < left side. < pressure, constriction < hot drinks < warmth. > warm applications > menstrual flow.

Keynotes

Climacteric ailments.
Hot flushes and perspiration.
Left-sided and move to right.
Sensitive to touch.
Sleeps into aggravation, worse after sleep.
Purplish lesions.

Ledum

Source	Marsh tea (wild rosemary).
Uses	Rheumatic conditions. Twitching muscles. Tetanus.
Eyes	Aching eyes. Extravasation of blood into skin. Black eyes.
Extremities	Gouty pains of foot. Joints, especially small joints. Swollen hot and pale. Rheumatism begins in lower limbs and ascends. Soles of feet painful.
Modalities	Better from cold. Putting feet in cold water. Worse at night and from warmth of bed.

Lycopodium

Source	Club moss.
Uses	A major polychrest. Many uses but affinity to disorders of urinary and digestive tract. Typically described as lean and sallow with a worried look. Intellectually keen but physically weak.
Mind	Melancholy. Fears being alone but dislikes people in same room. Irritable. Apprehensive (cf. Arg. nit., Arsenicum, Silica).
Head	Pressing headache on vertex. Worse from 4 to 8 p.m. Tearing pain in occiput, better for fresh air. Furrows in forehead.
Nose	Acute sense of smell.
Face	Greyish colour. Worried frown. Blue circles around eyes.
Throat	Stitches on swallowing. Better for warm drinks. Suppuration of tonsils beginning on right side.
Stomach	Dyspepsia from cabbage and beans. Desires sweet things. Pressure in stomach after eating only small amount. Burning eructations. Likes foot and drink hot.
Abdomen	Bloated after small meal. Liverish.
Stool	Diarrhoea or ineffectual hard stool. Painful haemorrhoids.
Urine	Pain in back. Heavy red sediment.
Respiratory	Cough with salty expectoration. Night cough. Rattly chest in infants.

Extremities	Right-sided sciatica. Cramps in calves.
Skin	Acne. Brown spots on face and abdomen.
Modalities	Worse right side < from above downward 4–8 p.m. < heat of room < warm applications except for throat and stomach. > motion > after midnight > warm food and drink > being uncovered.

Keynotes

4 to 8 p.m. modality.
< Cold drinks.
Flatulence after few mouthfuls.
Red sand in urine.

Mag. phos.

Source	Magnesium phosphate crystals.
Uses	Present in many body tissues. Affinity with nervous and muscular tissue causing neuralgic pains and spasm.
Mind	Laments about pain.
Eyes	Supraorbital pains relieved by warmth.
Mouth	Toothache, better for heat and hot liquids.
Abdomen	Colic causing patient to bend double. Relieved by rubbing, warmth and pressure. Belching produces no relief. Bloated sensation in abdomen.
Female	Menstrual colic.
Heart	Angina
Fever	Chilly, chills run up and down back.
Extremities	Cramps in calves.
Modalities	< right side < cold < touch. > warmth > bending double > pressure.

Keynotes

Right-sided.
Lightning pains.
Cramping.
Dread of cold.
Colic.

Mercurius

Source	Mercury.
Uses	Effects on all tissues, especially glands, bone and skin.
Mind	Weak memory. Slow answering questions. Weary.
Head	One sided tearing pain. Alopecia.
Eyes	Thick offensive profuse burning discharges.
Ears	Thick discharge.
Nose	Discharge. Ulceration of mucosa.
Face	Pale, earthy, dirty looking skin.
Mouth	Metallic taste. Spongy gums. Thick flabby tongue with impression of teeth. Odour.
Throat	Putrid. Ulcers and inflammation. Quinsy.
Stomach	Thirst for cold drinks. Continuous hunger.
Stool	Bloody and slimy, worse at night.
Genitalia	Irritating and itchy lesions.
Respiratory	Cough, cannot lie on right side.
Extremities	Dry skin. Profuse perspiration. Ulcers. Itching worse from warmth.
Fever	Chilliness, but worse from warmth, cold or damp.
Modalities	< night < wet < damp weather < warm room or bed.

Keynotes

Pains worse at night.
Perspiration does not relieve.
Flabby tongue with teeth imprint.
Bloody slimy stool.
Offensive discharge.

It is no surprise to find that mercurius is an antisyphilitic remedy and was used allopathically for that purpose in years gone by.

Nat. mur.

Source	A polychrest, common salt in potentized form.
Uses	Found in all tissues. Rheumatics, intermittent fevers and weakness.
Mind	Ill effects of grief and anger when related remedy ignatia fails to act. Depressed. Consolation aggravates. Irritable about trifles. 'Nice to know, difficult to live with'.
Head	Blinding headache, after menses and from sunrise to sunset. Schoolgirl headache, nervous, discouraged. Chronic semilateral migrainous headache, preceded by numbness and tingling in lips, tongue and nose. Relieved by sleep.
Eyes	Bruised with headache. Muscles weak and stiff. Conjunctivitis, burning and acrid discharge.
Nose	Coryza. Thin watery discharge. Loss of smell and taste.
Face	Oily, shiny skin with earthy complexion.
Mouth	Eruptions around corner of mouth. Mapped tongue.
Stomach	Hungry. Unquenchable thirst. Craves salt, averse to bread and slimy foods like oysters and fats.
Respiratory	Cough with stitching pain in chest.
Heart	Tachycardia. Chest feels constricted.
Extremities	Pain in low back, needs support. Arms and legs feel weak. Hangnails. Numbness and tingling.
Skin	Oily and greasy, especially hairy parts. Dry eruptions at scalp margin. Crusty eruptions in flextures. Eczema red-raw and inflamed. Worse on eating salt and at seashore.
Fever	Chill between 9 and 11 a.m.
Modalities	< noise < music < warm room < lying down < 10 a.m. < seashore. > open air > cold bathing > going without regular meals.

Keynotes

Emaciation, while living well.
Headache worse sunrise to sunset.
Headache preceded by blindness.
Mapped tongue.
Craves salt.
Worse at 10 a.m.

Nux vomica

Source	Poison nut plant. Use of dried seeds. Said by Boericke to be the 'greatest of all polychrests'.
Uses	A major polychrest, used for conditions of modern life. Affecting thin, nervous, irritable types. Mental strain in sedentary life.
Mind	Very irritable and sensitive to all impressions. Cannot bear noises, odours and lights. Dislikes being touched. Fault-finding and sullen.
Headache	Headache in occiput with vertigo. Intoxicated feeling. Worse in morning, after mental exertion, tea, coffee and alcohol. Frontal headache with desire to press against something.
Eyes	Photophobia worse in morning.
Nose	Stuffy colds after exposure to dry cold atmosphere. Blocked nose at night and odours.
Throat	Rough, scraped feeling.
Stomach	Nausea in morning after eating. Weight and pain in stomach after eating. Nausea and vomiting. Stomach sensitive to pressure. Loves fats and tolerates them. Dyspepsia from drinking coffee.
Abdomen	Flatulent dyspepsia with colic.
Stool	Constipation with ineffectual urging. Frequent ineffectual desire, passing small quantities at each attempt. Itching haemorrhoids. Diarrhoea after debauch.
Urine	Ineffectual urging. Strangury.
Male	Easily excited. Orchitis.
Female	Menses too early, too long, irregular. Dysmenorrhoea.
Respiratory	Asthma with fullness in stomach. Oppressed breathing.
Back	Lumbar pain. Burning in spine.
Sleep	Cannot sleep after 3 a.m.; awakes feeling awful.
Modalities	< morning < mental exertion < after eating < after spices, stimulants, < dry weather and cold. > sleep > evening > damp wet weather > strong pressure.

Keynotes

Quarrelsome, malicious, spiteful.
Thin, irritable and nervous.
Oversensitive to external impressions.
Covered during fever.
Chilly.
Wakes at 3–4 a.m.

Phosphorus

Source	Potentized from yellow phosphorus.
Uses	Affects mucous membranes and nervous tissue and haemopoietic tissues and liver.
Mind	Fearfulness. Tendency to start. Artistic, clairvoyant. Sensitive to external impressions. Fears death. Excitable.
Head	Burning pains. Brain fag.
Eyes	Fatigue of eyes. Green halo about candlelight. Long eyelashes.
Nose	Bleeding after menses. Oversensitive smell.
Face	Pale, sickly complexion.
Mouth	Gums bleed easily. Smooth, dry, red tongue. Burning in oesophagus. Thirst for large volumes of cold water.
Stomach	Hunger soon after eating. Belching. Craves water, vomits as soon as it warms in stomach. Pain in stomach relieved by cold water and ices.
Abdomen	Weak, empty, gone sensation. Congested liver. Jaundice.
Stool	Fetid stool and wind. Painless debilitating diarrhoea. Great weakness after stool. Rectal bleeding. Haemorrhoids.
Urine	Haematuria.
Female	Menses prolonged. Suppuration of breasts.
Respiratory	Hoarseness. Sore larynx. Violent tickling in throat while speaking. Aphonia. Cough worse from cold air, reading, laughing and talking. Tightness in chest. Oppressed breathing. Rusty sputum. Haemoptysis.
Back	Heat between shoulder blades.
Extremities	Ascending motor and sensory paralysis. Can lie only on right side. Arms and legs numb.

Fever	Chilly but lacks thirst.
Skin	Wounds bleed easily. Purpura, petechiae.
Modalities	< touch < physical or mental exertion < warm food or drink < change in weather < evening < during thunderstorm. > in dark > lying on right side > cold.

Keynotes

Tall, slender types with blonde or reddish hair.
Oversensitive.
Burning.
Weak, empty sensation.
Diarrhoea as if anus remained open.
Worse lying on left side.

Pulsatilla

Source	From pulsatilla nigricans, the Pasque flower.
Uses	The mental state is the main guide. Predominantly a female remedy.
Mind	Changeable, contradictory. Mild and yielding. Weeps easily. Full of fears of being alone, ghosts, dark. Likes comfort. Dread of opposite sex. Emotional. Mentally an April day.
Head	Frontal pains, particularly right temporal region, with lacrimation on affected side. Headache from overwork.
Eyes	Thick yellow bland discharges. Lids agglutinated. Styes.
Ears	Otorrhoea.
Nose	Catarrh, thick, bland and yellow.
Mouth	Dry mouth without thirst. Toothache relieved by cold water in mouth. Alterations of taste.
Stomach	Averse to fatty food, warm food and drink. Dislikes butter. Flatulence. Thirstlessness. Pain in stomach an hour after eating food.
Urine	Increased desire, worse when lying down.
Female	Amenorrhoea. Too late, thick, dark and clotted. Pain in back and feeling tired.
Male	Orchitis. Yellow discharge from urethra. Prostatitis.

Respiratory	Dry cough in evening; sitting up relieves it. Thick, bland expectoration.
Sleep	Sleeps on back, arms above head. Unrefreshing sleep.
Extremeties	Restless and chilly. Pains shift rapidly.
Skin	Urticaria and measles.
Fever	Chilliness without thirst. Chilly in spots. External heat is intolerable.
Modalities	< heat < rich food and fats < after eating < warm room. > open air > motion > cold applications and drinks though not thirsty.

Keynotes

Weeps easily.
Scanty menses.
Changing symptoms.
Rapidly changing pains.
Thirstlessness.
Dislikes fats.

Rhus toxicodendron

Source	Poison ivy.
Uses	Principally affects skin, mucous membranes and connective tissue.
Mind	Restless, with continued change of position. Listless and sad. Apprehension at night, cannot stay in bed.
Head	Heavy.
Eyes	Orbital cellulitis. Pustular eruptions. Ulceration of cornea. Iritis.
Stomach	Desire for milk.
Respiratory	Dry cough during chill.
Back	Pain and stiffness in small of back, better for motion and lying on something.
Extremities	Hot painful swelling of joints. Pains tearing in tendons, ligaments and fasciae. Limbs stiff and paralyzed.

	Sensitive to cold air. Sciatica worse in cold damp weather and at night.
Fever	Restless and trembling.
Skin	Red, swollen, intense itching. Vesicles, herpes, urticaria. Cellulitis.
Modalities	< sleep < cold, damp, wet, rainy weather < after rain < during rest
	> warm dry weather > motion > rubbing > change of position.

Keynotes

Restlessness, cannot remain still.
Sensitive to open air.
Triangular tip of tongue, red.
Vesicular eruptions.
Joints relieved by motion.
Worse for cold damp wet weather.

Ruta

Source	Rue (ruta graveolens).
Uses	Principally acts on periosteum and cartilage, flexor tendons. Parts feel bruised.
Eyes	Eye strain followed by headache. Weary while reading.
Back	Backache better for pressure and lying on it.
Extremeties	Limbs feel bruised. Pain and stiffness in hands and wrists. Tendons sore. Hamstrings feel shortened. Thigh pains when stretching the limbs.
Modalities	< lying < cold wet weather.

Keynotes

Eyes burn and ache and feel strained.

Sepia

Source	Inky juice of cuttlefish.
Uses	Predominantly a female remedy. Emotional and menopausal symptoms. Extremely chilly.
Mind	Indifferent to loved ones. Averse to family. Irritable and easily offended. Dreads being alone. Sad and weepy. Weeps when telling symptoms.
Head	Pain in shocks, worse at menses. Hair falls out.
Nose	Thick green discharge. Yellow saddle across nose.
Ears	Herpes behind ears and on nape of neck.
Stomach	Feeling of emptiness, not relieved by eating. Nausea at smell or sight of food. Tobacco dyspepsia. Nausea in morning before eating. Craves vinegar, acids and pickles. Loathes fat and worse after milk.
Abdomen	Flatulent. Liver sore and painful. Brown spots on abdomen.
Rectum	Feeling of ball in rectum. Constipation, large hard stool. Prolapse. Pain shoots up rectum and vagina.
Female	Bearing-down sensation, must cross limbs to prevent protrusion. Leukorrhoea. Menses too late and scanty or early and profuse. Prolapse of uterus and vagina.
Respiratory	Cough, dyspnoea worse after sleep.
Back	Weakness in small of back.
Extremeties	Restlessness in all limbs.
Skin	Itching not relieved by scratching. Chloasma. Urticaria in open air, better in warm room. Lentigo in younger women.
Modalities	< afternoon and evenings < washing and dampness < cold air < before thunderstorm. > exercise > warmth of bed > pressure > heat > after sleep.

Keynotes

Great sadness and weeping.
Indifference.
Pressure and bearing-down.
Flushes at climacteric.

Silica

Source	Pure flint.
Uses	Imperfect assimilation of tissues, debility. Diseases of bones, tissues. Useful in chronic infection and scars. Chilly.
Mind	Faint-hearted and anxious. Sensitive to all impressions. Headstrong children.
Head	Headache from fasting. Better warm and wrapped up. Profuse sweat of head.
Eyes	Styes, ulcers of cornea.
Nose	Dry crusts, which bleed when loosened.
Throat	Pricking sensation. Swollen parotid glands.
Stomach	Averse to meat and warm food.
Rectum	Fistula-*in-ano*. Fissures with spasm of sphincter. Stool comes out with difficulty and recedes again (bashful stool). Constipation before and during menses.
Female	Icy coldness of whole body. Milky acrid leukorrhoea. Abscess of labia.
Respiratory	Mucopurulent sputum. Slow recovery after chest infection. Violent cough when lying. Thick, yellow, lumpy sputum.
Extremities	Sciatica. Disorders of fingernails, white spots. Icy cold feet. Offensive sweat.
Skin	Abscesses, boils and old fistulous ulcers. Cracks at end of fingers. Promotes expulsion of foreign bodies from tissue. Keloid growths.
Fever	Chilly, very sensitive to cold air.
Modalities	< new moon < in morning < damp < menses < lying down. > warmth > wrapping up > wet or humid weather.

Keynotes

Children with large heads and open sutures.
Inactivity of rectum.
Bashful stool.
Offensive sweat.
Ailments with pus formation.

Sulphur

Source	Flowers of sulphur.
Uses	A great polychrest. Antipsoric. Affinity for skin. When carefully selected remedies fail to help, sulphur may arouse the reactive powers.
Mind	Forgetful. Delusions, 'thinks rags are beautiful'. Busy all the time. Selfish and opinionated, no regard for others. Lazy. Irritable, depressed, thin and weak.
Head	Constant heat on top of head. Dry scalp.
Eyes	Burning, ulceration of margins. Ulceration of cornea.
Nose	Red and scabby.
Lips	Bright red and burning.
Stomach	Food tastes too salty. Drinks much, eats little. Milk disagrees. Desires sweets. Acidity with eructations. Weak and faint about 11 a.m., must have something to eat.
Abdomen	Internal rawness. Sensitive to pressure.
Rectum	Itching and burning of anus with redness. Morning diarrhoea, painless, drives out of bed.
Urine	Enuresis. Frequency at night. Urgency with burning.
Female	Vagina burns. Thick, black menses causing soreness. Nipples cracked.
Respiratory	Difficult respiration; wants window open. Rattling of mucus. Oppression of chest. Dyspnoea in middle of night.
Extremities	Hot sweaty hands. Burning in hands and soles at night. Offensive sweat.
Sleep	Cannot sleep between 2 and 5 a.m.
Skin	Dry, scaly, unhealthy. Every little injury suppurates. Itching, burning, worse for scratching and washing. Itch after warmth.
Modalities	< at rest < when standing < warmth of bed < washing and bathing < in morning < 11 a.m. < alcohol < periodically. > dry warm weather > lying on right side > drawing up affected limbs.

Keynotes

Cannot stand, aggravates symptoms.
Dirty, filthy people cannot bear washing.
Relapsing complaints; sensation of burning.
11 a.m. Aggravation.
Diarrhoea in early morning.
Painful discharges.
Red anus.

Thuja

Source	Thuja occidentalis, (Arbor vitae).
Uses	Acts on skin, gastrointestinal tract, genito-urinary organs and brain. Corresponds with Hahnemann's sycotic conditions.
Mind	Fixed ideas, strange person at side, soul and body separated, something alive in abdomen. Emotionally sensitive, music makes them weep.
Head	Pain like a nail being driven through. Neuralgia from tea. White scaly dandruff. Greasy skin of face.
Eyes	Ciliary neuralgia. Eyelids agglutinated. Styes. Inflammation of sclera and iris.
Nose	Thick discharge, green mucus and pus.
Mouth	Tip of tongue painful. Tooth decay.
Stomach	Loss of appetite, averse to fresh meat and potatoes. Cannot eat onions. Tea-drinking dyspepsia.
Abdomen	Distended. Brown spots. Constipation with rectal pain. Anus fissured with warts.
Urinary	Severe cutting after micturition. Frequency. Urgency.
Male	Gonorrhoea. Induration of testes. Prostatic enlargement.
Female	Sore and sensitive vagina. Warty growths. Leukorrhoea. Polypi.
Respiratory	Asthma in children.
Extremities	Feels as if limbs made of wood or glass and would break easily. Pain in heels.
Skin	Polyps, warts, naevi and ano-genital ulcers. Sweet strong perspiration. Dry skin, brown spots. Eruptions on covered parts. Sensitive to touch.

Sleep	Insomnia.
Fever	Sweat on uncovered parts.
Modalities	< at night < from heat of bed < at 3 a.m. and 3 p.m. < cold damp air < after breakfast and after fat and coffee. > left side drawing up limbs.

Keynotes

Fleshy, dark, unhealthy skin.
Fixed ideas.
Large granulations around eyes.
Bashful stool (silica, sanicula).
Diarrhoea.
Dirty skin with brown spots.
Sweat on uncovered parts.
Legs feel as if made of wood or glass.
Sycotic conditions.

29

The nosodes

Nosodes are medicines derived from human or diseased tissue, e.g. pus, discharges. As with all remedies, they are attenuated in the preparation and by the process of potentization no active tissue is present in the medicine. There are approximately 200 nosodes available from a wide range of sources.

There are two distinct groups of nosode; those for which there is a distinct symptom picture and which have been fully proved, and those with a limited symptom picture.

The first group contains the familiar nosodes:

1. Tuberculinum.
2. Medorrhinum.
3. Syphilinum.
4. Psorinum.
5. Carcinosin.

The second group contains those remedies used for prophylaxis or as a follow-up after the patient has had a specific illness. Based on the similimum, the remedy has been prescribed.

1. Rubella nosode.
2. Influenzinum.
3. Cocksackie nosode.
4. Diphtherinum.
5. Pertussin.
6. Morbillinum.
7. Parotidinum.
8. Acne bacillus.

There are many others in this group and a fuller list of available nosodes can be obtained from the manufacturers.

Potencies of other related nosodes include allergens, such as:

1. House dust mite.
2. Cat fur.
3. Horse dander.

4. Mixed-grass pollen.
5. Timothy grass.
6. Moulds.

Again, the manufacturers can provide a list. In some unusual cases where you have identified an agent causing the disease it may be possible for the manufacturer to make up a potentized medicine for you.

Nosodes are prescribed when the symptom picture is clear for a particular remedy, or where a patient has complained of never being well since a particular illness. This can be of use in many cases such as viral fatigue, or the malaise associated with glandular fever.

Nosodes tend to be prescribed infrequently or as a single dose. The potency can vary but 30C or 10M as a single dose is a standard regime.

Isodes

The use of tissue, whether diseased or healthy, taken from the patient is called *isotherapy*.

Sarcodes

Sarcodes are homoeopathic remedies prepared from the healthy tissues of animals. Their affinity with the corresponding organ in humans is used as a basis for therapy. A specific branch of this, *organotherapy*, is used extensively in France.

Bowel nosodes

These will be described more fully later in this chapter.

Tuberculinum

Source	A nosode from tubercular abscesses.
Uses	Useful in chronic renal problems. Lax fibroid individuals with slow recovery from ill health. Always tired. Symptoms always changing. Great liability to catch colds. Emaciation. Consider when there is a family history of tuberculosis.
Mentals	Contradictory symptoms. Excitement and melancholy, insomnia and stupor. Depressed on wakening.

	Fear of animals, especially dogs. Temper tantrums. Desires change. Always on the move.
Head	Intense neuralgias. Iron band around head.
Ears	Offensive discharge. Perforation of drums.
Stomach	Averse to meat. All-gone hungry sensation. Desires cold milk.
Abdomen	Early-morning offensive diarrhoea.
Female	Profuse early menses. Dysmenorrhoea. Benign mammary tumours.
Respiratory	Enlarged tonsils. Desires cold air. Hard hacking cough.
Skin	Chronic eczema. Worse at night.
Modalities	< motion < music < before a storm < damp < draught < after a sleep. > open air

Keynotes

Tall, thin, blue eyes, fair.
Narrow chest.
Family history of tuberculosis.
Changing symptoms.
Takes cold easily.
Rapid emaciation.
When best selected remedy fails to act.

Syphilinum

Source	A nosode of syphilitic pus.
Uses	Chronic disease. Shifting rheumatic pains. Susceptibility to ulceration and abscesses.
Mind	Loss of memory. Apathy. Feels as if going insane. Fear of night. Hopeless. Despair. Obsessive behaviour, repeating words or washing hands.
Head	Falling of hair. Neuralgic headache causing sleeplessness and delirium.
Eyes	Chronic inflammation of cornea. Photophobia. Pain at night. Ptosis.

Mouth	Teeth decay, and serrated teeth. Excessive saliva runs out of mouth at night.
Stomach	Craves alcohol.
Extremities	Sciatica, worse at night. Rheumatism around shoulder joint and deltoid. Indolent ulcers. Repetitive hand washing.
Female	Profuse leukorrhoea.
Skin	Reddish brown eruption.
Modalities	< night < sundown to sunrise < seashore < in summer. > inland > mountains.

Keynotes

Pain from darkness to daylight.
All symptoms worse at night.
Profuse leukorrhoea.
Falling of hair.
Craving alcohol.

Medorrhinum

Source	Gonococcal pus (sycotic remedy).
Uses	Deep-acting. Chronic ailments. Chronic thick yellow discharges. Chronic rheumatism. Irritability of nervous system.
Mentals	Weak memory; times passes too slowly. Poor concentration. Fears insanity and the dark. Melancholy with suicidal ideas. Chronic fatigue. Impatient and restless. Starts easily. In a hurry to do things.
Head	Burning pains worse in occiput. Worse from jarring. Itching of scalp, dandruff.
Face	Small boils, worse during menses.
Mouth	Thick grey mucus.
Stomach	Ravenous hunger after eating. Thirst. Craves salt, sweets and warm things.
Stool	Intense itching and needle-like pains in rectum.

Urine	Pain in renal areas. Renal colic. Nocturnal enuresis.
Female	Profuse dark menses. Genital warts. Sterility. Severe menstrual colic. Cold breasts, sore to touch.
Male	Urethritis. Urging and painful micturition.
Respiratory	Asthma. Sore larynx. Dry cough, worse at night. Better lying on stomach.
Extremities	Back pain, burning. Spine sore to touch. Rheumatic pains in shoulders, extending to fingers. Relieved by motion. Soreness of soles. Restless and fidgety legs.
Skin	Yellow. Intense itching. Tumours and abnormal growths.
Modalities	< when thinking of ailment < daylight to sunset < heat < inland. > seashore > lying on stomach > damp weather.

Keynotes

Weakness, physical and mental.
Cannot speak without weeping.
Cravings.
Urinary symptoms.
Rheumatic pains, burning.
Trembling all over.

Psorinum

Source	Scabies vesicle.
Uses	Psoric problems. Debility. Skin conditions. discharges.
Mind	Hopeless despair. Suicidal tendency.
Head	Chronic headaches. Worse for change of weather.
Eyes	Recurrent eye infections.
Ear	Oozing scabs around ears. Offensive discharge from ears. Intolerable itching.
Face	Eruptions on face.
Throat	Offensive saliva. Quinsy.
Stomach	Always hungry.

Stool	Bloody and fetid.
Respiratory	Asthma with dyspnoea. Hay fever. (Single dose before season starts is said to be useful.)
Skin	Dirty. Dry hair. Intolerable itch. Herpetic eruptions, worse from warmth of bed. Slow-healing ulcers. Oily skin.
Modalities	< coffee < change of weather < cold or least draught of air. > heat, warm clothing (even in warm weather).

Keynotes

Filthy smell.
Sensitive to cold air.
Offensive discharges.
Always hungry.
Quinsy.
Asthma.
Hay fever.

Carcinosin

Source	Originally breast epithelium. (Other tumours have been used.)
Uses	Family history of cancer, tuberculosis, diabetes. Past history of glandular fever or vaccination reaction. When strongly indicated remedy fails to act.
Mind	Dullness of mind, anticipatory anxiety. Fastidious, or the opposite! Insomnia.
Head	Throbbing pains.
Eyes	Blue sclerotics.
Skin	Café-au-lait complexion. Pigmented naevi. Eczema.
Modalities	< afternoon.

Keynotes

Symptoms alternate in laterality.
Sensitive to either heat or cold.

The bowel nosodes

The bowel nosodes were first described by Paterson[1] and Bach (pronounced Batch, subsequently of flower remedy fame). In 1936 a paper described their work, ‘The potentised drug and its action on the bowel flora’. This paper reviewed their findings on 12 000 cases.

They noted that non-lactose-fermenting bacilli were found in 25% of stool specimens. The appearance of the particular organism related to a particular homoeopathic remedy that the patient had previously been taking.

The fact that the stool yielded organisms not usually found in normal stool led them to conclude that the homoeopathic remedy had altered the bowel flora, as there was a definite delay in their appearance after taking therapy. The pathogenic organism found in the stool was a result of the remedy’s action on the patient.

Paterson and Bach found that each of the organisms correlated well with a particular symptom picture. They stated that:

1. The specific organism is related to the disease.
2. The specific organism is related to the remedy.
3. The homoeopathic remedy is related to the disease.

Paterson offered a symptom picture, based on clinical observations of sick people.

Bowel nosodes are used infrequently by many homoeopaths; however they are useful in certain cases.[1]

A list of the main remedies and recommendations for use is given below.

Morgan (Bach)

This is used for the most commonly found organism.

Congestion is the keynote.

Head	Congestive headaches, flushed face. < heat, excitement, travelling.
Mentals	Introspective, anxious and apprehensive about health. Avoids company, but nervous alone. Depression with suicidal tendency.
Gastro-intestinal tract	Congestion of mucosa, reflux, bitter taste. Congestion of liver, bilious attacks with headache > vomiting.
Respiratory	Congestion of nasal and bronchial mucosa. Recurrent pnuemonia.

Genito-urinary	Congestive headache with menstrual onset, with congestive dysmenorrhoea and flushing.
Circulation	Congestion characterized by varicose veins and piles, blueness and sluggish circulation.
Joints	Congestion affecting knee joints and phalanges.
Skin	Morgan Bach for congestion of skin with itching < heat. Good for children (refer: Sulphur, Psorinum, Graphites and Petroleum).

There are two subtypes of bacillus Morgan – *pure* and *Gaertner.*

Pure	Used where there is marked skin eruption, or disturbance of liver. Related remedy: Sulphur.
Gaertner	More useful in acute attacks of liver, e.g. cholecystitis. Also for acute renal colic. 4–8 p.m. periodicity. Related remedy: Lycopodium.

For Morgan Bach the related remedies are sulphur, calc. carb. and lycopodium.

Proteus

Suddenness is the keynote. Symptoms secondary to nervous system.

Mentals	Violent temper, emotional hysteria and epileptiform seizures.
Circulation	Spasm, such as dead fingers of Raynaud's, intermittent claudication, angina and Ménière's disease.
Digestive	Ulcers, sudden onset due to stress.
Muscular	Cramps of muscles.
Skin	Sudden-onset angioedema, sensitivity to ultraviolet light.

Related remedies to consider: Apis (skin), Ignatia (mental), Nat. mur. (digestive), Cuprum met. (muscles).

Gaertner

Malnutrition is the keyword.

Mentals	Hypersensitive child, overactive brain with undernourished body.

Digestion	Inability to digest food properly. Emaciation and wasting disease.

Related remedies: Phosphorus, Silica and Merc. viv.

Dysentery co

Keywords **nervous tension, anticipatory in nature**.

Mentals	Tension, anticipatory anxiety, sensitive to criticism, fidgets, even choreic movements. Tension headaches at regular intervals 7–14 days.
Digestive	Spasm of plyorus. Acute pain in stomach > vomiting. Ulcer symptoms brought on by prolonged mental strain.
Cardiovascular	Palpitations before events.

Related remedies: Argentum nit., Arsenicum alb. and Kalmia.

Sycotic co

Non-lactose-fermenting coccus. Keynote is **irritability**.

Mentals	Nervous, irritable, twitchy, fear of dark. Twitching of face and eye muscles.
Head	Irritation of sinuses.
Digestive	Irritation of whole gastrointestinal tract. Acute or chronic gastroenteritis. Loose stool. Urgent diarrhoea, worse after eating.
Respiratory	Acute or chronic catarrh. Enlarged tonsils and adenoids.
Circulation	Anaemia.
Neuromuscular	Rheumatic aches, worse for damp.
Genito-urinary	Marked action on urinary tract causing irritation or membranes resulting in cystitis, urethretis, vulvo-vaginitis. Leukorrhoea and pain in tubes and ovaries.

Prescribing bowel nosodes

Paterson[1] recommends strict prescribing rules. The remedies are deep-acting. A full case history is needed.

If a specific remedy is found, use it, but if the choice lies between related remedies then a bowel nosode may be used. For example, if the picture lies between sulphur, calc. carb. and graphites, then Morgan pure may be the choice.

The stronger the mentals, the higher the potency. Conversely, the more pathological the symptoms, the lower the potency.

A single high-dose potency is sometimes recommended, accompanied by more frequent low-dose related remedies.

Old cases that have received homoeopathic remedies in the past may best be treated by low potency and not repeated too often, i.e. less than 3 months between doses.

References and further reading

1. Paterson J. *The Bowel Nosodes*. Supplement in *Allen's Key Notes* (Allen HC.) pp. 387–402. New Delhi: B Jain Publishers, 1988.
2. Boericke W. *Pocket Manual of Homoeopathic Materia Medica* (ninth edn). New Delhi: B Jain Publishers, 1988.
3. Allen HC. *Allen's Key Notes* (eighth edn). New Delhi: B Jain Publishers, 1988.
4. Gibson. *Studies of Homoeopathic Remedies*. Beaconsfield: Beaconsfield Publishers, 1987.
5. Tyler ML. *Homoeopathic Drug Pictures*. New Delhi: B Jain Publishers, 1987 (reprint).
6. Blackie M. *Classical Homoeopathy*. Beaconsfiled: Beaconsfield Publishers, 1986.
7. Laing R. Using the bowel nosodes. *Br Hom J* 1995; **84**(1): 21–25.

Appendix 1: useful books and addresses

History and philosophy

Bannerjee PN. *Chronic Disease: Its Cause and Cure.* New Delhi: B Jain Publishers, 1988.
Blackie M. *Classical Homoeopathy.* Beaconsfield: Beaconsfield Publishers, 1986.
Cook T. *Samuel Hahnemann. His Life and Times.* Wellingborough: Thorsons, 1971.
Hahnemann S. *Organon of Medicine.* (translation Kunzli *et al.*) London: Victor Gollancz, 1992.
Kent JT. *Lectures on Homoeopathic Philosophy.* New Delhi: B Jain Publishers, 1991.
Kent JT. *Repertory of Homoeopathic Materia Medica.* Sittingbourne: Homoeopathic Book Service, 1993.
Roberts H. *The Principles and Art of Cure by Homoeopathy.* New Delhi: B Jain Publishers, 1988 (reprint).
Ruthven-Mitchell G. *Homoeopathy.* London: W.H. Allen, 1975.
Speight P. *A Comparison of Chronic Miasms.* Budsworthy: Devon Homoeopathic Group, 1986.

Materia medica

Allen HC. *Allen's Keynotes.* (eighth edn) New Delhi: B Jain Publishers, 1988.
Boericke W. *Pocket Manual of Homoeopathic Materia Medica.* (ninth edn) New Delhi: B Jain Publishers, 1988.
Gibson D. *Studies of Homoeopathic Remedies.* Beaconsfield: Beaconsfield Publishers, 1987.
Tyler M. *Homoeopathic Drug Pictures.* New Delhi: B Jain Publishers, 1988 (reprint).

Treatment

Borland D. *Children's Types*. London: British Homoeopathic Association, 1950.
Clarke JH. *The Prescriber*. New Delhi: B Jain Publishers, 1988.
Gemmell D. *Everyday Homoeopathy*. Beaconsfield: Beaconsfield Publishers, 1987.
Herscu P. *Homoeopathic Treatment of Children*. Berkeley, CA: North Atlantic Books, 1991.
Pratt N. *Homoeopathic Prescribing*. Beaconsfield: Beaconsfield Publishers, 1985 (revised edn).

Introductory text

Lockie A. *A Family Guide to Homoeopathy*. London: Book Club Associates (Courtsey of Hamish Hamilton), 1991.

Useful addresses

Faculty of Homoeopathy
The Royal London Homoeopathic Hospital
Great Ormond St
London WC1N 3HR

British Homoeopathic Association
27a Devonshire St
London W1 1RJ

Society of Homoeopaths
2 Artisan Road
Northampton NN1 4HU

The British Institute of Homoeopathy
Cygnet House
Market Square
Staines
Middlesex TW18 4RH

Appendix 2: case histories

One of the comments I hear most frequently from those interested in introducing homoeopathy into practice is that there is just not the time to do so.

I have sympathy with this view, as the workload in primary care is ever-increasing. However, I believe it is possible to introduce homoeopathy even at a basic level and to incorporate it into practice using a variety of prescribing techniques.

The skills come with experience, an understanding of fundamental homoeopathic principles, a thorough knowledge of materia medica and knowing your way around the repertory.

In this appendix different cases and different approaches are described, demonstrating the styles that can be used. At this point I repeat, as throughout this book, that there are no short cuts. You have to work hard and build up a skill base to practise effectively.

Think how to approach a case at different levels. In many consultations you develop a sense of whether you are dealing with an acute problem that may only require a simple prescription. In others there are deeper underlying factors where a quick prescription would be inappropriate and a constitutional or miasmatic approach may be needed. These patients need a lot more time. Some more radical colleagues have criticized my approach: I am not treating the underlying problem and may be only palliating a case. Although this may be true, I have had to compromise between lack of time and the realization that a substantial number of patients want homoeopathic treatment on the National Health Service, as they cannot afford private fees. Both I and my patients accept this constraint.

However, even in long cases it is possible to manage time effectively. If a patient presents as a difficult case, I give out a detailed homoeopathic questionnaire with specific instructions on how to complete it. Primary care notes contain an extensive background on a patient which may obviate the need to probe a history as much as if a patient were new to you. The notes should contain details of past illness, family and social history.

Different approaches are described below. Start with simple problems and build up a repertoire of remedies as your confidence and experience grow.

Case 1

Mr AC, a 44-year-old man, sprained his ankle whilst playing football with his son. On examination there was no bony tenderness, but the left lateral ligament was bruised and swollen.

Advice was given regarding rest, icepacks and elevation. Arnica 30C every 15–30 min was advised for the first 2 h, then half-hourly thereafter for 24 h.

He required no other analgesia.

Discussion

This is an example of the use of a specific remedy. Many cases in practice are like this. A specific remedy – arnica for bruising, aconite for shock – can be given as a first-line response.

Case 2

Mrs AS, aged 36, presented complaining of acute onset of flu-like symptoms. She had shivers, mild temperature and generalized muscle aches.

She was given aconite 6C repeatedly every 15 min with little improvement. In view of the generalized shakes and severe muscle pains she was give gelsemium 6C half-hourly, which caused a diminution of her symptoms.

Discussion

Although not typical, I use a variety of flu remedies such as aconite, ferrum phos., gelsemium and occasionally pyrogen for these symptoms. I think they are a good example of an epidemic remedy. Many people may present over a few days with a similar picture and it may be worthwhile considering these remedies.

Case 3

Mr FJ, a 47-year-old, presented with a 3-month history of general malaise, inability to concentrate and fatigue on exertion.

He had confirmed glandular fever at the time with a positive monospot test.

In his past history there was little of note, but his family history revealed a strong history of carcinoma and diabetes mellitus.

Discussion

This combination of symptoms, family history and 'never well since' suggested the use of carcinosin 1M. This was unsuccessful and after 2 months he was given glandular fever nosode 10M. Over the next 3 months his symptoms slowly improved, though not completely. His mental symptoms improved first; this is a good sign that the remedy was having an effect.

This is an example of a 'never well since' remedy and is useful when a provoking factor can be identified.

Case 4

Mr AL, aged 34, presented with a short history of 3 weeks of generalized rheumatic symptoms.

There was no precipitant and all his investigations were normal, including erythrocyte sedimentation rate, viscosity and rheumatoid factor. There was no other history.

His joint pains were mainly affecting the small joints of the hands and feet. They were worse with rest and eased by movement.

He preferred warm weather and found his symptoms were worse for damp and wet weather.

Based on this limited information and the time constraints of general practice, he was given Rhus tox. 6C three times daily until his symptoms improved.

After 1 week his symptoms had cleared.

Discussion

This would be considered an example of keynote prescribing where key symptoms led to the choice of a remedy that fits the picture. If this patient had not improved I would have considered looking for a constitutional remedy.

Case 5

Mrs SK, a 46-year-old shop worker, was seen complaining of a 3-week history of abdominal pain, cramps and diarrhoea.

For 2 years she had complained of attacks of morning diarrhoea and hypogastric cramps following an attack of what she described as food poisoning after eating shellfish.

Subsequently she complained of panic attacks, which she described as a sensation of tingling all over her body, palpitations and flushing of her skin. These would occur after an attack of diarrhoea.

Any unusual symptoms would result in an attack of diarrhoea and panic.

She described herself as 'one big knot of fear'.

Garlic, onions and alcohol exacerbated her symptoms.

Past medical history

1985	Panic attacks
1991	Laparotomy for gangrenous omentum

Family history

Brother	Died age 48 of carcinoma of the stomach 3 years earlier
Sister	TB as a child
Sister	TB as a child

Social history

Nil of note
Works as a shop worker in a very hectic job. Very stressful

Homoeopathic history

Appearance
Fair, overweight. Pale brown eyes
Medium build: 5′ 4″ (approx. 1.60 m)
Weight: 70 kg
Smartly dressed. All clothes matched

Manner
Relaxed, but underlying tension. Frowning
Wriggling her hands

Generals

Heat. Likes heat and warm weather

Cold. Very chilly. Dislikes cold. Feels cold easily

Activity. Always on the go. Cannot sit still. Has to do something

Desires/aversions. Hates fat, butter, milk. Could vomit at sight of fat

Sleep. Needs little sleep, but always tired

Energy. Has lots of energy, but then flags after couple of hours and feels useless

Particulars
Head. Associated right-sided throbbing headache with some attacks

Urinary. Profuse flow of clear urine during attack

Skin. Red blotchy rash over face and neck during attack

Mentals
Worries all the time about her health, disease and her illness

Fears. Death
Her illness
Cancer
Dark in late evening and being alone at night

Likes company, better for people being around
Likes sympathy and reassurance
Extremely tidy. Does not like anything out of place

Dreams – recurrent, of teeth falling out
Intolerant and irritable but bottles it up, especially if things not going as she would like

Physical

BP	140/80 mmHg
CVS	NAD
RS	NAD
GIT	NAD

Investigations
Stool culture, sigmoidoscopy and barium enema all negative

Diagnosis

Anxiety state/panic attacks

Rubrics (page in Kent's repertory)

Fear of death	p 44
Fear of own ill health	p 7
Anticipatory fear	p 45
Fear of being alone	p 43
Aversion to fats	p 480
Likes company	p 12
Skin, mottled red with anxiety	p 1309

Remedy choice

I graded the symptoms above as the most significant.

After repertorization the clear choice was between phosphorus and arsenicum album. The clear choice to me was arsenicum. I visited this woman in her home and the house was spotlessly clean and she was obsessively tidy. She was restless despite being in her own surroundings and admitted to being always 'on the go'.

She was full of fears and anxiety with a strong aversion to fats. Phosphorus types tolerate or like fats. Her abdominal symptoms do not describe the typical burning sensations of arsenicum, but overall I felt that constitutionally she was a typical arsenicum.

Management

After much discussion and reassurance the patient was prescribed Arsenicum album 200C three doses daily on day 1. She was asked to monitor her symptoms and their frequency.

She was reviewed 6 weeks later as I felt that this remedy would take some time to produce improvements. She reported a lessening in her anxiety and bowel symptoms sufficient to make her life more tolerable. She was advised to take a further dose of Ars. alb. 200C and repeat monthly only if there was no further improvement.

A final review 4 months after the initial consultation revealed that she was living a much more normal life and had not needed any further treatment at that stage.

Discussion

This is a classical long case. The prescription chosen was a constitutional remedy. This is the typical approach to a homoeopathic case, taking all the details in a single session. However primary care is a setting which may allow some of the history to be taken over a series of shorter consultations, when the patient is already known.

Index